Praise for *The Curl Revolution*

"Growing up, this book would have empowered me to appreciate my curls at an earlier age. There are so many voices that tell us who to be and what to love and this book will stand out among them. What a beautiful illustration of embracing and loving who you are! It makes my heart happy to be a part of something that will uplift and celebrate all who have curly crowns! CURL POWER!"

—**JORDIN SPARKS,** singer

"With NaturallyCurly, Michelle Breyer created the first online resource that addressed curly hair textures. Michelle did an excellent job of creating a community for people who have been largely ignored."

—**JOHN PAUL DEJORIA,** cofounder, Paul Mitchell hair products and Patrón Spirits Company, philanthropist, entrepreneur

"NaturallyCurly is my FIRST source for all things curly, wavy, kinky, coiled and textured. When I started think about building HAIRiette—my own hair care line—it was, far and away, the most comprehensive source online, hands down. What I love most about NaturallyCurly is their ability to embrace everyone with texture. They've got a great team and Michelle has become a dear friend in my curly world. I am grateful for their steadfast commitment to women (and, ahem, men) with curls!"

—**TANYA WRIGHT,** actress *Orange Is the New Black* and *True Blood*

"NaturallyCurly has been an incredible advocate of the natural hair movement. It has given curly-haired women a platform."

—**RICHELIEU DENNIS,** cofounder, Sundial Brands (makers of SheaMoisture)

"The texture revolution happened because of the world wide web and NaturallyCurly."

—**ANTHONY DICKEY,** curl expert and author of *Hair Rules*

"Those of us with curly, kinky, and coily hair have often been rendered invisible, easily divisible, or marginal by the mainstream beauty industry. *The Curl Revolution* disrupts the notion of a straight rigid standard and centers the lens on a mighty and diverse dynamic community made of individuals where no two curls are the same. It expands images and the collective imagination."

—**...HAELA ANGELA DAVIS,** image activist

THE

Curl

REVOLUTION

THE

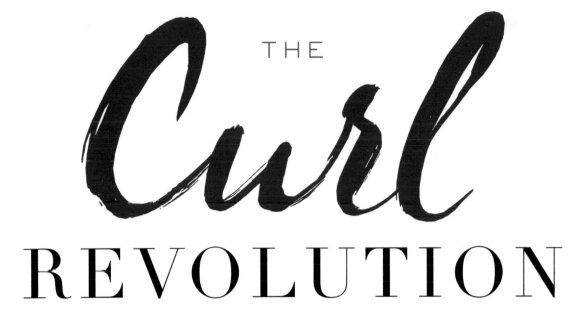

Curl

REVOLUTION

Inspiring Stories and Practical Advice
from the **NaturallyCurly** Community

MICHELLE BREYER

with contributions from Erica Metzger and Gretchen Heber

PHOTOGRAPHY BY KARSTON "SKINNY" TANNIS

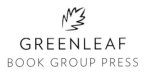

GREENLEAF
BOOK GROUP PRESS

Published by Greenleaf Book Group Press
Austin, Texas
www.gbgpress.com

Distributed by Greenleaf Book Group

For ordering information or special discounts for bulk purchases, please contact
Greenleaf Book Group at PO Box 91869, Austin, TX 78709, 512.891.6100.

Design and composition by Greenleaf Book Group
Cover design by Greenleaf Book Group
All photographs are copyright Karston Tannis except the following: Taliah Waajid (10)
photo credit: James Hogan; Patrice Yursik (20) photo credit: Steve Yursik; Lisa Sugar
(31) photo credit: Maria Del Rio; various (72, 86, 183) photo credit: Getty Images;
Maria Thompson (139) photo credit: Keith Clayton; Pintura (180) photo credit: Mike
Marshall, Rhea Carter (181) photo credit: Rhea Carter; Asia Brazil (188) photo credit:
James Hogan; and Graham (224) photo credit: Graham.

Cataloging-in-Publication data is available.

Print ISBN: 978-1-62634-428-0

eBook ISBN: 978-1-62634-429-7

Part of the Tree Neutral® program, which offsets the number of
trees consumed in the production and printing of this book by
taking proactive steps, such as planting trees in direct proportion
to the number of trees used: www.treeneutral.com

Printed in China on acid-free paper

17 18 19 20 21 22   10 9 8 7 6 5 4 3 2 1

First Edition

CONTENTS

PREFACE. ix

1: THE CURL REVOLUTION 1

2: LIVING THE CURLY LIFE—Why Curly Hair Isn't Just Hair . . 21

3: TEXTURE TYPING—It's More than Just Curl Pattern 41

CURL PATTERN GUIDE 53

4: CREATING YOUR CURLY REGIMEN—What Products
to Use When 73

5: CURL KABOBS TO PLOPPING—Tried-and-True Curl
Styling Techniques 95

6: GOING NATURAL—Transitioning, the Big Chop,
and Everything In Between 129

7: CUTTING CURLS—Unlocking the Potential of Your Texture . . . 159

8: COLORING CURLS—A Rainbow of Options 175

9: CURL CHALLENGES AND THEIR SOLUTIONS 189

10: CURLY KIDS—Where It All Starts 205

11: CURLY MEN—Not Just a Buzz Cut 219

CONCLUSION 227

ACKNOWLEDGMENTS 229

CURLIPEDIA 231

INDEX 243

ABOUT THE AUTHOR 249

ABOUT THE PHOTOGRAPHER 251

PREFACE

When NaturallyCurly launched in 1998, we had no idea we would be an integral part of a huge grassroots movement that would transform the way society views curly hair.

In the beginning, we juggled our day jobs at the newspaper and our growing families—four children were born in the first four years—with a fledgling hobby that was becoming a business. As the company grew and we hired new employees and added new sites, it was hard to get a true sense of all the ways the world was changing—of how we were helping to change the world.

Over the years, there were many times when we considered compiling some of the best tips and stories from our website into a book. But to do a book that would truly reflect the power of Naturally-Curly—and be worthy of the many other people who have helped shape the curly world—would take time and resources. Time was always in short supply. Every day there was so much that needed to be done—clients to call, stories to write, products to sell. And there were always meetings—lots of meetings.

In numerous conversations over the past year—with other industry pioneers, influencers, and curly girls—the idea for the book kept bubbling to the surface.

There came a point where it could not be ignored. This book had to happen. We had to make the time.

Having been a part of the curl revolution since the beginning—before there was a curly world—I have a unique perspective. I've had the good fortune to work closely with so many of the pioneers in this important category.

Because NaturallyCurly has no single point of view, but provides information about all techniques, philosophies and product offerings, I've learned that this isn't a one-size-fits-all industry.

Our community represents a wide range of ethnicities, age groups, and hair textures from around the world. The diversity of our readers has given me an appreciation for the wide range of hair concerns and curl journeys.

In *The Curl Revolution: Inspiring Stories and Practical Advice from the NaturallyCurly Community*, we have compiled some of the best information from NaturallyCurly's experts and community members collected over the past two decades. We will take you through every step of the curl experience, from figuring out your texture type to figuring out your ideal regimen to finding the right cuts and styles.

But this information—these tips—is only a part of the picture. We also wanted to share the inspirational stories of some of the top curly entrepreneurs, stylists, influencers, and community members, without whom there would be no Curl Revolution.

While we feature many curl icons, including actresses and singers, we didn't want to fill a book with studio shots of glamorous models. We wanted our book to showcase beautiful photos of real curly women, men,

We hope this book serves as a starting point for you. The NaturallyCurly network is a living, breathing organism with millions of visits each month. We hope you'll visit often to discover amazing content, share your own stories and tips, get advice, and find inspiration. Throughout this book you will see this icon which directs you to NaturallyCurly.com to discover even more empowering and engaging content.

and children—students and teachers, social workers, and accountants. Many started their curly journey on NaturallyCurly.

This book celebrates the inspiration, empowerment, and education that transformed the curl landscape. It's a way of saying thank you to the many people who have been a part of this journey to create change.

Perhaps most of all, this book is a tribute to the amazing, loyal, and passionate community that is NaturallyCurly. They are the reason why this revolution has happened. Their collective voices have been a powerful force in the Curl Revolution.

We thank you, and we love you.

—*MICHELLE BREYER,*
cofounder of NaturallyCurly

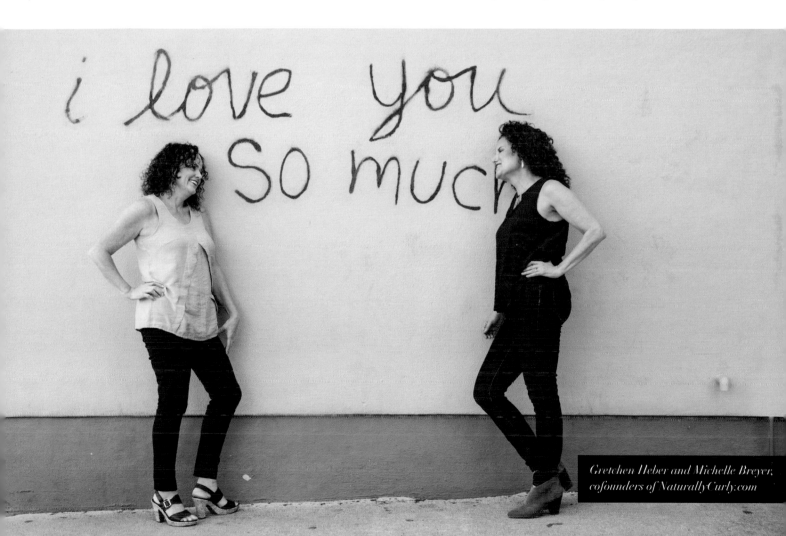

Gretchen Heber and Michelle Breyer,
cofounders of NaturallyCurly.com

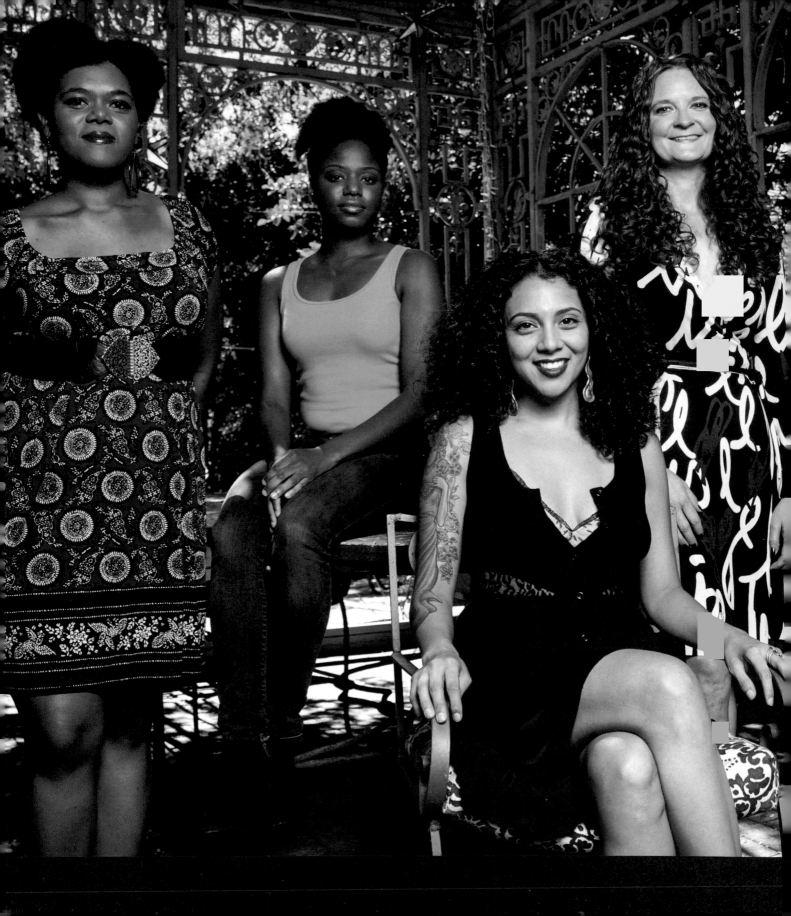

Chapter 1

THE CURL REVOLUTION

*I*t was a Sunday morning in the spring of 1998. Three friends and fellow journalists (Gretchen Heber, Lori Hawkins, and me) were gathered at a coworker's house for brunch. We were in the midst of one of our regular, lengthy bitch sessions about our curly hair, lamenting the perils of the Austin humidity and longing for the sleek haircuts we had always wanted but could never have.

These were lonely times for the curly girls of the world. It was as if waves, curls, and coils didn't exist. This was the era before Facebook, before blogs, before Instagram, before YouTube. Influencers and meet-ups didn't really exist. Google had just launched.

An eavesdropping techie friend was mesmerized by our discussion.

"Do you talk about your hair all the time?" he asked.

"Pretty much," we said with a laugh.

"You should start a magazine or a website or something about curly hair," he suggested.

The three of us looked at each other. Maybe it was the mimosas we had been drinking all morning or our collective lifetimes of frustration at being curly girls in a straight-haired world, but something clicked.

We went to the nearest computer and did a search for meaningful information about curly hair. Not surprisingly, we found only one web site; it touted one of the few existing product lines specifically for curly hair. While it was a nice site, it provided limited information for people hungry for advice about how to care for their curls. It reinforced what we had known all our lives. The world had all but ignored the sixty-plus percent of the population with curls, coils, and waves.

The idea for a curly website took shape, and we ran with it.

Over the next few months, we sketched ideas and enlisted a neighbor's 14-year-old son to design our site. Wanting to differentiate ourselves from the curly perms of the '80s, we dubbed our site NaturallyCurly.com, to make it clear this was for people whose hair is naturally curly, coily, or wavy. We based our logo design on the cartoon character Frieda, Charlie Brown's friend who—at every opportunity—showed off her naturally curly hair. Our young web designer found a way to animate the logo's curls, a feature we were thrilled with.

From day one our goal was to create a place for people like us—a forum to provide support, tips, and inspiration for other curlies. In short order, the heart of the site became CurlTalk, a discussion forum where curlies could continue the type of conversation that had galvanized us to launch the site.

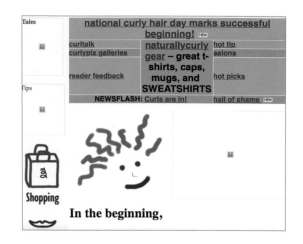

We always talked in terms of texture type, styles, or concerns, but never ethnicity. We built the website on a hunch that we weren't the only ones who figured if we were frustrated with our hair, there were sure to be others out there—we found out quickly that we were right.

As for our business plan, we really didn't have one. We thought we might sell a few T-shirts emblazoned with our logo. But NaturallyCurly wasn't conceived as a moneymaking venture. It was a way to provide a sorely missing resource and sense of community to other curlies. That was it.

When we launched the site in September 1998, we watched excitedly as the visit count grew. Hundreds of daily visits quickly became thousands. People from countries

> "The biggest change is people have access to information and affirmation. Women can be aspirational with each other. It's such a huge change—you don't have to figure it out by yourself. There's a whole community that's figuring it out with you."

—Jamyla Benu, founder of Oyin Handmade hair care line

Texture: 4a, high porosity, fine, medium density

Regimen: My Wash 'n Go is my go-to style. I use Oyin Juices & Berries, Moisture Dew, and Shine and Define for definition and styling with Oyin Handmade Pudding on top to seal it.

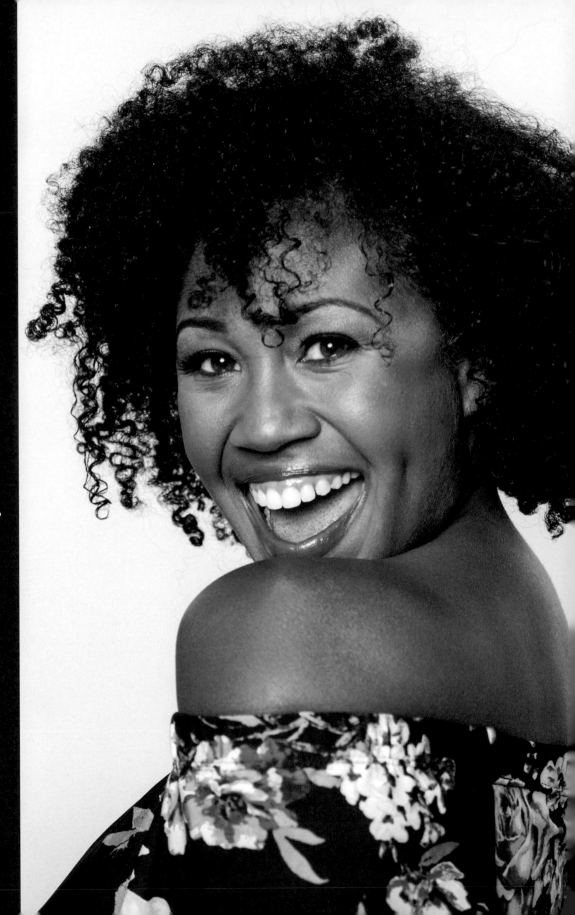

> "It all happened in one day. I was working on an episode of *24*, wearing a straight, spikey wig. I decided one day that I no longer wanted to wear a wig; I wanted to wear my own hair. The hair person asked the executive producer to come over, and I asked him if I could wear my own hair. He said, 'Why didn't you always wear it that way?' That was the end of that. I'll be wearing my hair the way it grows out of my head."

—Tanya Wright, actress (*Orange Is the New Black*, *True Blood*), entrepreneur, author, creator of HAIRiette

Texture: 3c, high porosity, fine, thick

Regimen: I co-wash once a week with HAIRiette Co-Wash and style with HAIRiette Curl Crème. I seal the ends with HAIRiette Oil Blend. I like it better on the 3rd or 4th day.

around the globe—from Australia to Brazil to Israel—discovered NaturallyCurly.

CurlTalk, a discussion forum we created for curlies to share ideas and advice, became the heart of the site. "Curlversations," such as the one that launched the idea for the site, became indispensable for most of our members, who admittedly spent hours chatting with their NaturallyCurly curlfriends.

People not only found us, but they also came back over and over. They told their friends about us. CurlTalk discussions soon grew beyond hair topics to every subject imaginable—from TV shows to politics to boyfriend troubles—as our readers became a community. CurlTalkers coordinated "Curl Gatherings" in their cities to meet each other—an early incarnation of the meet-ups to come. Swap boards were created to trade products.

"NaturallyCurly saved my life," jokes hair care marketing veteran Tauri Laws-Phillips, who transitioned after 16 years of relaxing. "I would read all the articles and go home and try them. It helped me relearn who I was."

We received excited emails from our readers. They shared their curl struggles and insecurities, which we posted on the site. They shared stories of transitioning from relaxed to natural hair at a time when it was still resisted by husbands, parents, grandparents, and others in their communities. We heard heartbreaking stories of kids being teased for their hair and of teenage girls trying to fit in with their straight-haired peers. Depending on their texture and their backgrounds, they faced different obstacles. But they all shared a desire to embrace their texture and they wanted to help each other. They also learned that texture transcends ethnicity.

"When I found NaturallyCurly's Curl-Talk in 2006, I discovered there was this whole community that didn't just include black women, but also white women with their own struggles," says Patrice Yursik, founder of the *Afrobella* natural hair blog. "That was a real eye-opener to me. It made me realize this was more of a universal struggle than I thought it was."

Their voices—coming together from around the world, from all different backgrounds—started to reshape the conversation.

"NaturallyCurly was the first site I went on when I was researching all things curly," recalls actress and entrepreneur Tanya Wright, who has appeared in such shows *Orange is the New Black* and *True Blood*.

"What I specifically liked was that it embraced texture instead of ethnicity. It embraced everyone."

We had our share of detractors. There were people who believed dedicating a site to curly hair was crazy. "It's just hair!" was a refrain we heard fairly often. Some just couldn't understand how a head of curls or coils could have such a powerful impact on a person's self esteem. But we knew there were plenty of people who did understand and that we were doing something important, even necessary.

Every time we approached curly girls on the street, or in an airport, or on a subway to compliment their hair and tell them about the site, you could see their face light up and an instant kinship formed. Within minutes, we'd launch into meaningful conversations about our curly journeys—the horrible nicknames, bad haircuts, lack of products, regular trips to the salon for relaxers, and the family members who pressured us to straighten our natural tresses.

Occasionally through the years women recognized and approached us to tell us how NaturallyCurly changed their lives. They found a stylist on NaturallyCurly who changed their life by finally giving them a good haircut. Or perhaps, they discovered their "Holy Grail" products on the site. For many, NaturallyCurly was the place that finally gave them the courage to transition from a relaxer to their natural hair, despite a society that told them their natural hair texture was somehow inferior—"bad hair."

I remember one New York Curl Gathering in particular. A woman approached me and tentatively showed me her employee badge. The photo—a woman with hair pulled tightly back in a severe bun—looked nothing like the confident, curly woman who stood in front of me. She told me that for 50 years, she had hated her curly hair and had done everything she could to hide it. But finding NaturallyCurly had changed that for her by providing the tools and support she needed to embrace her curls. She cried as she told me her story, and I cried along with her.

More than one person in the industry has called us "The United Nations of Curls" because we were the one place providing a wide range of viewpoints, whether it be wet versus dry cutting, to "'poo" or not to "'poo," the benefits and drawbacks of silicones, or the different ways to transition from relaxed to natural hair. NaturallyCurly provides information on all cutting techniques, textures, hair care brands, and points of view. Our goal has always been to provide accurate information

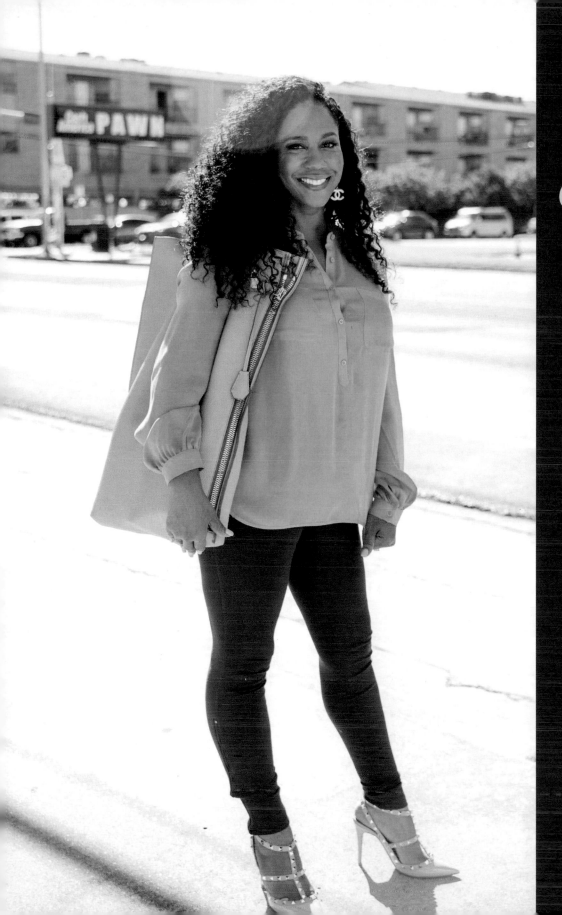

" I started my company before the birth of natural products, when there weren't many options. I was a newly natural mother looking for natural products. If a product doesn't exist and you're smart, you bring something new to the market. That's why I launched CURLS."

—Mahisha Dellinger, founder of CURLS product line

Texture: 3b/3c, low porosity, fine, thick

Regimen: Co-wash once a week on Wednesdays with CURLS Blueberry Bliss Reparative Hair Mask. I do a full wash on Saturdays with CURLS Blueberry Bliss Reparative Hair Wash and Mask. I also will use Blueberry Bills Reparative Leave-in Conditioner followed with CURLS Blueberry Bliss Curl Control Jelly. In the winter, I use CURLS Twist & Shout Cream.

> " It didn't start with manufacturers and stylists. It started with the people who said our hair texture isn't bad, it's beautiful."

—Anthony Dickey, author, stylist, and founder of Hair Rules Salon and hair care brand

Texture: 4a, medium porosity, coarse, thick

Regimen: Rinse with water. Cleanse with Hair Rules Cleansing Cream, once a month. If it's longer, I put in a little Kinky-Curly Curling Cream.

with which women with curls, coils, or waves can make their own choices. The beautiful thing is that we now have choices, and we can make informed decisions.

"NaturallyCurly was the Bible," says Janell Stephens, who created the popular Camille Rose Naturals hair care line in 2011. "I spent hours on NaturallyCurly."

NaturallyCurly has served as a unifying force at a time when there has been so much division. Some questioned whether a site created by three Caucasian women could serve the needs of those of other ethnicities. Some felt that any mention of relaxers or a flat iron should be grounds for banishment from the site. But, with open hearts and open minds, we persisted in the belief that texture is a unifying topic rather than one of division.

At the end of the day, we want nothing more than for people to feel good about themselves, whether they embrace their natural texture or straighten their curls, no matter their texture type. NaturallyCurly is a place free of judgment.

Early on, articles about NaturallyCurly appeared in publications such as *People* magazine, *USA Today,* and *Glamour. Nightline* did a segment on NaturallyCurly and our passionate community. To many reporters we were an odd, amusing curiosity. They couldn't imagine that a group of people could dedicate so much time and energy to curly hair.

We never dreamed that NaturallyCurly would become the first and loudest voice of a revolution—the place where brands would be created and launched, top influencers would develop their followings, and millions of curly lives would be changed. But NaturallyCurly became the epicenter of a powerful grass-roots movement.

"The texture revolution happened because of the World Wide Web and NaturallyCurly," says curl expert Anthony Dickey, author of *Hair Rules* and founder of a salon and a product line of the same name. "It spread like wildfire. It allowed people to have a place to speak without interruption—their stories, their pain."

From California kitchens to salons in Atlanta, in communities around the world, creative entrepreneurs and renegade stylists have slowly changed the way people think about curls and coils.

When Taliah Waajid's mother refused to let her relax her hair, she learned to manage, style, and love her natural hair without the use of chemicals. Her natural hairstyles attracted requests from friends and neighbors for her services. At the age of 14 she started her hair care business working out of

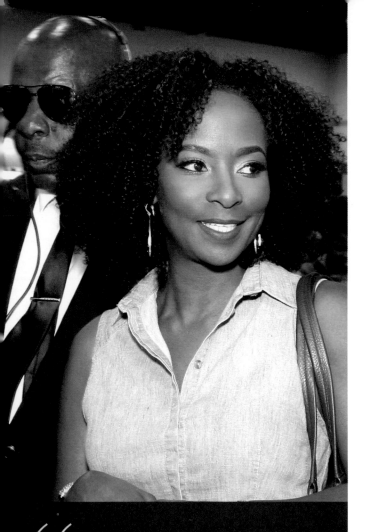

her home. She opened her first natural hair salon in 1988 in Harlem.

Taliah moved to Atlanta, Georgia, opened a natural hair salon, and in 1996 launched Black Earth Products—the first complete line of hair care products formulated for natural hair and locs. A year later she created the first gathering dedicated to natural hair—the World Natural Hair, Health, and Beauty Show. The show, which started with just 50 exhibitors and barely 100 attendees, has grown into a massive two-day event attracting over 200 exhibitors and 30,000 attendees from around the world.

Taliah says her decision to promote other brands has been about providing the consumer with choices. "I wanted women to know that they had a choice. I wanted them to know that it was a healthier choice that was just as beautiful as wearing straight hair. Most women I met did not know that."

Pioneer Ouidad, a curl stylist in New York, opened a salon catering to curly hair in 1984. Everyone from beauty editors to bankers told her she was crazy. And yet, her eponymous salon has persevered as a successful testament to the power of curls.

"Did I think curly hair would be so big? Yes," says Ouidad. "Did I think the industry would wrap its arms around it? Not so much. That's

That's kudos to NaturallyCurly and everyone else. Deep in my gut, I knew there were so many people like me."

Diane Bailey, a four-decade texture expert, changed the focus of her Tendrils Salon in Brooklyn to natural hair in 1991.

"I couldn't stand the smell when I opened a jar of relaxer. One day I decided that was the last day I'm putting a relaxer in someone's hair," Bailey says. "My mother thought I was going to go broke. I lost some clients, but some of them stayed. They were in for the journey."

Mixtress Lisa Price was concocting products in her Brooklyn kitchen in a venture that would become Carol's Daughter, which she launched in 1993. She says it's been interesting to watch the Curl Revolution happen, and to be a part of it.

"It was as if all hair care was dependent on relaxers or a hot comb," Price says. "You had to figure out a way around it. We were cocktailing with the few things we could find. There was so much to explore because there was nothing available."

Richelieu Dennis and his childhood friend Nyema Tubman created products using the recipes of Dennis's grandmother and sold them on the sidewalks of Harlem.

That was how SheaMoisture was born. These curl-centric product lines have become go-to standards for curly women everywhere.

In lower Manhattan, Lorraine Massey opened Devachan Salon. She felt the industry wasn't meeting the needs of wavy and curly women and developed a dry cutting technique that now is used by thousands of Deva-trained stylists. The DevaCurl line of products, which was one of the first to promote sulfate-free shampoos and styling products without silicones, grew out of the salon. "No 'pooing" has become a part of the curly lexicon, and most brands now offer a sulfate-free option.

Sisters Titi and Miko Branch started Curve Salon in Brooklyn with one thing in mind: to respond to the unmet needs of texture in all of its forms. Because they couldn't find the products they needed for their clients, they used their grandmother's recipes to create the puddings and custards that are the core of the very successful Miss Jessie's line.

To the north in Toronto, veteran stylist Jonathan Torch developed an obsession with curly hair after botching a curly client's cut. He embarked on a personal mission to master the art of cutting and caring for curly hair, studying how curly hair shrinks, what makes it frizz, and how texture patterns differed on

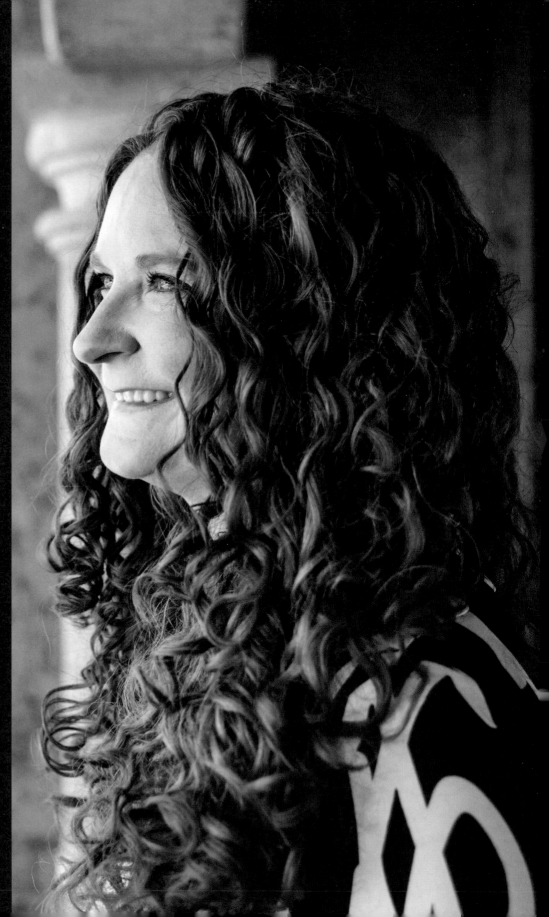

"I was experimenting with products, but my hair was still horizontal. One day I found a random recipe for flaxseed on the Internet. I tweaked it for a week, adding aloe and jojoba oil. I went to CurlTalk and said 'I cracked the code!' I got 30 emails from people wanting to buy it. I printed labels and taped them on the bottles. That product was Jessicurl Rockin' Ringlets. That was 14 years ago and now we have 12 products."

**—Jessica McGuinty,
creator of Jessicurl products**

Texture Type: 3a, high porosity, coarse, thick

Regimen: After rinsing really well I condition in the shower with Jessicurl Too Shea! Extra Moisturizing Conditioner, or if my hair feels particularly dry that day, I'll use the Jessicurl Deep Treatment instead. While my hair is still soaking wet (and still upside down) I put a quarter- sized dollop of Too Shea, and a puddle of Jessicurl Rockin' Ringlets into my palm, rub my hands together and rake that through. Then scrunch (with my head still upside down), then scrunch in a puddle of Jessicurl Spiralicious Styling Gel.

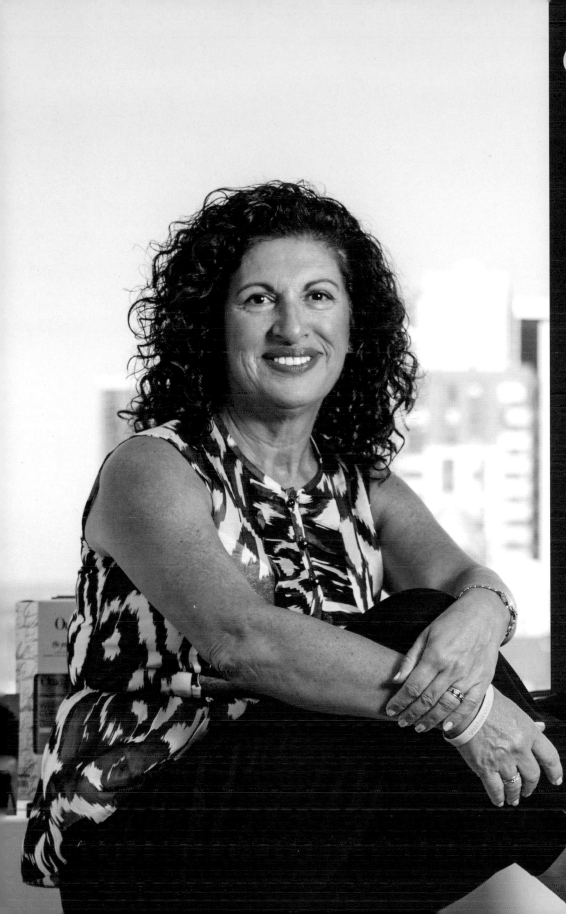

> " I came from Lebanon. When I came here, it blew my mind. In the United States—the greatest country because we're so multicultural—I thought I would see everything. All I saw were people following the rules. Everybody had straight, blonde hair. It was a uniform."

—Ouidad, "Queen of Curls," founder of Ouidad Salon, the first curly salon, and creator of the Ouidad product line

Texture: 3a, medium porosity, fine, medium density

Regimen: Day 1, I always shampoo hair using Climate Control Shampoo and Climate Control Conditioner. I add a little Deep Treatment Curl Restoration Therapy as a styling aid to seal the cuticle and "rake and shake" with Ouidad Climate Control Heat & Humidity Gel, putting clips at the roots for volume, and let it dry naturally. I spray a little Ouidad Finishing Mist.

> " In the beginning days, it started with frustration. And then the conversation began. Little conversations turned into bigger conversations. Everyone added their own spin. It wasn't just one singular voice."

—Miko Branch, cofounder of Miss Jessie's product line

Texture: 3b, medium porosity, coarse, thick

Regimen: I use Miss Jessie's Leave-in Condish and Jelly Soft Curls, and wash once a week with Miss Jessie's Crème de la Curl Cleansing Cream. I deep condition with Super Sweet Sweetback Treatment

each head. This obsession was the impetus of his Curl Keeper line of products.

In the case of personal trainer Jessica McGuinty, a regular on NaturallyCurly's CurlTalk, a quest to create the perfect gel for her own use turned into Jessicurl, a popular line of curl products.

"I typed 'curly hair' into Google in 2001, and NaturallyCurly.com popped up," recalls McGuinty, who had been called names like Chia Pet, Egghead, and Brillo Pad as a teenager. I thought, 'These are my people!'"

"A flaxseed gel recipe shared by McGuinty on CurlTalk morphed into Jessicurl's Rockin' Ringlets Styling Potion, the first of 12 products now sold around the world.

There are too many pioneers to mention; they could fill a book. While they traveled different paths, they all were driven by their own experiences and a passion to make the world better for people with curls and coils. This entrepreneurial spirit exists today, with new hair care brands and influencers carving out their niche in the growing market.

We were blessed with good timing. We started at a time when society was becoming increasingly more accepting of our multiculturalism, and the standard of beauty was changing. Slowly we began to see more curls and coils on the catwalks, red carpets, and magazine covers.

Within a few years after launching, social media had dramatically changed the digital environment by empowering people to create their own web sites, blogs, and YouTube channels to share information about their hair. Many of these influencers were early CurlTalkers on the NaturallyCurly web site.

A sense of empowerment was growing, rippling well beyond NaturallyCurly. With the power of social media, people no longer had to wait for magazines or major hair care brands to notice them. They could create their own platforms and products and spread the word themselves. They gained power as people sought more authentic sources—people who looked like them and had gone through struggles similar to their own. An endorsement from a top blogger now carries more weight than a campaign featuring a major celebrity.

"I discovered CurlTalk in 2006 when I was struggling with my own curls in grad school," says Nikki Walton, who became an active CurlTalker with a big following. "I greatly enjoyed learning about my curls and teaching others."

She started her own blog, *CurlyNikki*, in 2008, one of the first, which continues to be among the most popular natural hair care blogs. Walton is an active partner in TextureMedia, and is a best-selling NAACP Image Award–nominated author and TV personality.

As word of the growing array of curl products spread on NaturallyCurly, it created demand for a place to buy them. To fill this need, we opened CurlMart (now called shop NaturallyCurly) in 2004. It was the first e-commerce site dedicated to products especially for curly hair, and it was a launchpad for many brands that are now curly household names.

"It was a no-brainer," says Mahisha Dellinger about launching her CURLS brand on NaturallyCurly. "I thought, 'If I'm launching, I have to launch on NaturallyCurly.' It was the most important way to reach our audience organically."

CURLS is now a staple in the curl category, with products available at retailers such as Target, Wal-Mart, and Sally Beauty.

Large beauty brands and media companies began to take notice of NaturallyCurly's large and passionate community and the growing number of products popping up in CurlMart.

But even though curls were getting attention, some brands continued to view us as a trend instead of a 365-days-a-year market.

I can't count the number of times over the years that large brands would say: "We're not focusing on curls this year."

Every time I heard that, I wanted to scream, "Our hair is not a campaign!"

For those of us with curls, our hair is something that affects our lives 365 days a year.

But with the powerful momentum created by this passionate consumer—a consumer who spends significantly more than their straight-haired friends—texture has now become a major focus for even the largest brands. Today nearly every brand—small and large—has products specifically for curly hair.

Watching these changes over the past 19 years, it's hard for me to remember what the world was like when I was growing up as a curly girl with a straight-haired mother and sister. In an attempt to manage my unruly locks, my mom kept my hair cut short in a pixie. I longed for a ponytail that swished.

We moved to California in the middle of my sixth-grade year. On my first day of school, cruel classmates at my new school teased me because they said I looked like a boy. In seventh grade, I dreaded going to my history class because several boys called me "Bozo." Every day, they sat behind me whispering that nickname.

In the eighth grade, I rebelled against my mom's insistence on the cropped cut. I grew out my hair. I discovered curling irons, plastic rollers, and hairspray and tried in vain to style my hair like Farrah Fawcett. Most of my friends at my San Jose high school had shiny, silky, straight manes that feathered effortlessly. On my birthday each year, my best friend would spend an hour with her brush and blow-dryer, trying to straighten my hair. The dryer was usually smoking by the end. We would plaster my 'do with Final Net and, for a day or two, I had hair that vaguely resembled that of my classmates. It felt like plastic, but I felt "normal."

Through the years of trying to manage my curls, I practically developed PTSD after all the bad haircuts from stylists who didn't understand that cutting curly hair requires different techniques from those used to cutting straight hair. They didn't understand the concept of shrinkage—that snipping two inches off a head of curls actually resulted in a loss of four inches or more in length.

As a young professional woman, my quest for products was just as frustrating. I could find products for dry, normal, and oily hair. There were product lines called "Long and Silky" and "Short and Sassy." But curlies like me were forced to make do, wading through a sea of products for all hair types except our own. We learned to layer different products together to get the look we wanted—a now widely used practice called "cocktailing."

Like many of you, I have tried everything to beat my curls into submission. I once accidentally got a "chemical haircut" in college when a stylist left the lye relaxer on too long and chunks of my hair broke off at the root.

Eventually I developed a long, tedious routine of blowing out my hair and then setting it with Clairol hot rollers. I dreaded any sign of humidity that would inevitably make me resemble the Saturday Night Live character Roseanne Roseannadanna.

This struggle continued into my late twenties, until I moved to Texas and had to accept humidity as a daily fact of life.

It was time to make peace with my curls.

I was lucky to find a stylist who helped me grow out my bangs and gave me a cut that worked with my curls. I can remember the trepidation I felt wearing my natural curls to work for the first time. My curl confidence grew a little each day, and I began to appreciate the unpredictable personality of my ringlets, although they still can frustrate me on a hot, humid day. I rarely go anywhere without a ponytail holder, just in case.

Over the years, I have been asked if texture is a trend. I've heard people say "Aren't you glad curls are in style?"

It's like telling people that their eye color is in fashion. Curls and coils are a basic part of who we are. That doesn't mean we can't straighten them if we want. It does mean that we no longer have to change them in order to be accepted or to be considered beautiful, professional, and sexy.

"To decide not to straighten my hair was freedom for me," says Daniela Gomes, a Brazilian journalist and activist in the country's black political movement, who wears a big, beautiful Afro. "I can be the person who I am—a professional, beautiful woman—and be natural. I can change my hair if I want to. But it will be *my* choice if I change."

Of course, there is still a long way to go. Plenty of people still think curls are a problem that requires fixing. Most stylists still leave cosmetology school without ever working on a curly head. According to DevaCurl—which provides curl training to stylists—there is only one curl-trained stylist for every 32,000 curly people in the United States.

There are the Patti Stangers of the world (the "Millionaire Matchmaker"), who make public comments such as "I like stylish, curly, wavy hair, but my millionaire men don't."

There are still plenty of stories of kids being kicked out of ballet class because their coils don't fit the preferred image, and people who feel that they must straighten their hair to look "professional."

One woman recently blogged about a coworker telling her "You know, you might not have gotten the job if your hair was curly at that interview."

As I write this, a Kentucky high school has been forced to lift its ban on natural hairstyles like cornrows and twists after a social media uproar. Seriously? Well into the 21st century, we're still having to fight these battles?

With the Curl Revolution we choose to focus on the incredible progress that's been made since NaturallyCurly launched nearly two decades ago.

"I'd like to think any stigmas that did exist are going away," says Lisa Sugar, cofounder of PopSugar, a global lifestyle and media brand. "People are more open to all types of beauty."

Texture: 4a in some spots and 3c in other spots, high porosity, fine, thick

Regimen: L.O.C.: I use Carol's Daughter Hair Milk Cleansing Conditioner or Carol's Daughter Marula Curl Therapy Gentle Cream Cleanser, and once a month shampoo with Carol's Daughter Monoi Shampoo, or Carol's Daughter Monoi Conditioner, or Carol's Daughter Monoi Repairing Hair Masque. I use the Carol's Daughter Monoi Repairing Anti-Breakage Spray followed up with Carol's Daughter Monoi Oil Sacred Repairing Serum or pure Monoi oil, depending on what my hair is doing. My final step is Carol's Daughter Hair Milk Combing Cream.

> "The natural hair movement taught me about what was going on outside of myself. The issues might be different, but at the core of it there's a thread of similarity I'd never thought of before."

—Patrice Yursik, founder of *Afrobella*

Texture: 3c, medium porosity, fine, thick

Regimen: I use shampoo every 10 days. I co-wash if I need to, every 4 or 5 days. It depends on my level of activity. On weekends I try to deep condition and detangle my hair, always with a wide-tooth comb, working from tip to root. Then I typically use a spray-on leave in, then a creamy styling product, and finally a light oil. Brands I love include Oyin Handmade, Soultanicals, SheaMoisture, Hair Rules, Naturally Smitten, and Alikay Naturals. My hair LOVES Aussie 3 Minute Miracle conditioner.

Chapter 2

LIVING THE CURLY LIFE—
WHY CURLY HAIR ISN'T JUST HAIR

LETTER TO MY 10-YEAR-OLD SELF

Dear Zaria: Don't murder your hair! I know you like it straight and unnoticeable. I know you like the way it feels when it blows in the wind. But the way straightening destroys it, it's not worth it. Embrace your curls. Love them. You'll find that you get compliments everywhere you go. I know everyone else your age has straight hair. Be unique!"

—ZARIA SHARED THIS LETTER WITH HER STYLIST, ROBIN SJOGREN

Three-year-old Patrice Yursik was happily playing on the swing in her yard on the island of Trinidad. Her mom and sisters usually spent a lot of time carefully combing and braiding her long hair into two braids. But on this particular day, Yursik's hair was out and free. Inexplicably, a little girl came up to Yursik, braided her hair to the swing, and left her there, trapped.

"I was on the swing screaming and crying," recalls Yursik, founder of *Afrobella*. "My mom came and had to cut all my hair off and leave it in the swing."

Her long hair was gone and Yursik started kindergarten with a TWA—a teeny weenie Afro.

"I had a lot of trauma around that experience," Yursik said. "Washing and combing my hair became a big production. Hair became a big deal for me pretty early. Think of all that trauma we carry because of our experiences with our hair."

Gather a group of curlies, and you'll hear heartbreaking stories about the bullying they endured, the low self-esteem they suffered, and the desperate measures they took because of their hair. There's the frustration of having little control over your hair and the envy that comes with not fitting in with the accepted standard of beauty. Many have grown up being told they had "nappy" or "bad hair."

Living curly means having cabinets full of hair products yet still searching for your new Holy Grail. Curl pioneer Ouidad describes it well: "A straight-haired person is just a head of hair, where a curly-haired person is a head with a lifetime of experiences."

> **"Pretty much everything I did over the years was crazy, ridiculous, damaging, and a terrible waste of time, money, and tears: Ironing it with a clothes iron. Rolling it up in soup cans. All manner of perms and straighteners. Flat irons and crimpers. Salon haircuts."**
>
> **—AN ANONYMOUS CURLTALKER**

Jessica McGuinty's bad haircut before the summer of her freshman year of high school left indelible scars on her psyche.

"It was super short and people called me names like Liberace, Little Dutch Boy, Brillo Pad, and Chia Pet," says McGuinty. "When it grew out, it grew *out*."

To tame her hair, McGuinty would cut the legs off of a pair of nylons and sleep with the crotch on her head. "I woke up with an indentation on my head."

Most of the time, gaining curl confidence can be a journey—a process. If you've spent most of your life straightening and fighting your texture, you may not feel like yourself when you wear your hair in its natural curly or coily texture.

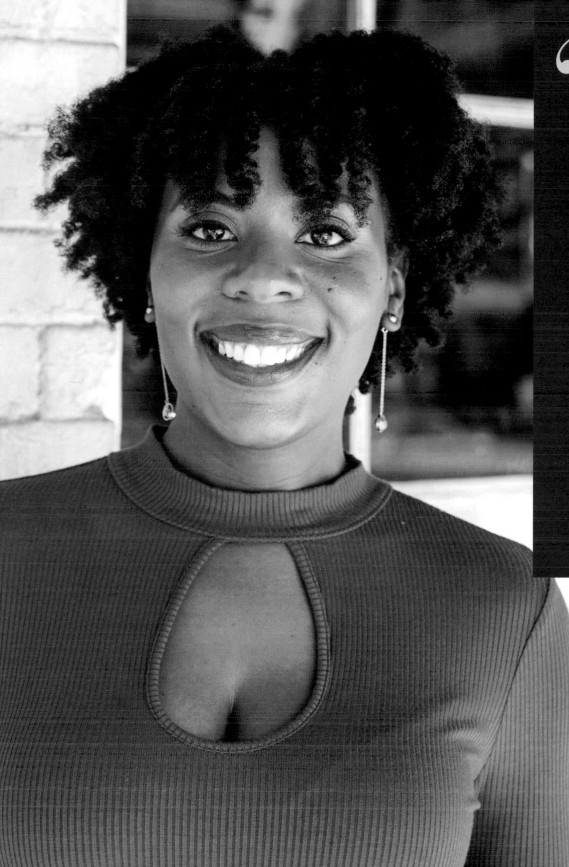

> "With natural hair you have to be more patient. I felt like when I wet my hair, it would be really, really curly. It was hair I didn't really know how to style until I did more research and discovered products that worked."

—Jamila Pope, employee of Texas Medicaid

Texture: 4c, high porosity, fine and coarse, thick

Regimen: I just figured it out. Since June, I've been using Design Essentials Coconut & Monoi Curl Refresher, Eden Bodyworks Coconut Shea Curl Defining Creme, and castor oil. When I want to moisturize it, I use the same products.

> **"** In the Dominican Republic, there are some girls who aren't even allowed to go to school with their hair curly. The norm of our community was getting blowouts. I was the only girl with curly hair. Had I grown up with what's going on now, I feel like my life would have been completely different."

**—Ada Rojas, founder of
Gypsy in the City blog**

Texture: 3b/3c, low porosity, fine, thick

Regimen: To style, I use Curly Hair Solutions Curl Keeper Frizz Control Gel, Leave-in. DevaCurl Super Cream, SheaMoisture Hibiscus & Coconut Curl Enhancing Smoothie or Design Essentials Curl Enhancing Mousse.

It's a struggle not made easier by pop culture, which still seems more comfortable with straight hair. In 2001, NaturallyCurly led a boycott of the Disney film *The Princess Diaries*. In the movie, the character played by actress Anne Hathaway gets a makeover to straighten her wild curls, so that she might appear more "royal." To us, the message was curl-hostile. You're not pretty enough or serious enough or, indeed, royal enough if you have curly hair. To be a princess, you must have straight hair—a negative message for the young, impressionable, curly girls who saw the movie.

At the time, a spokesperson for actress Julie Andrews (who plays Hathaway's grandmother, the queen), responded to our boycott by saying, "Sometimes girls with curly hair like to have straight hair. I'm sure Julie feels it wasn't done to offend anyone."

Entertainment Weekly joked that "Maybe a blow-dryer would straighten out this mess."

This was obviously written by a straight-haired editor who had never endured the teasing that most curly kids have experienced or the anxiety of heading out on a date fearing what humidity or rain would do to your hair.

Actress Toni Trucks says that since booking her first TV show in Los Angeles, her natural curls have been chopped off, dyed, and straightened.

"To date, I have only appeared on screen once with my curly hair," she says, referring to the look for her role in *Twilight Saga: Breaking Dawn—Part 2*.

Our curl journeys and struggles vary dramatically depending on where we grew up and the culture in which we grew up. For black women, going natural carries with it different challenges based on beauty standards going back generations.

"I bought into the belief that natural hair wasn't beautiful enough and straight hair was better," says Natasha Gaspard, founder of Mane Moves Media. "That was ingrained in me since I was little."

When she made the decision to go natural, she felt empowered. But it took time to redefine herself. "Once I accepted it, that was it."

In addition to finding the right products and styles, living the curly lifestyle very much affects what happens inside each of us. It can be a major shift in the way we see ourselves.

"I am constantly exposed to people commenting on and manipulating my hair, wishing it were straighter, curlier, *more* than what it is," Trucks says. "I have to actively fight against internalizing this kind of scrutiny,

CONTI PORTA

> " I always had a 'grass is greener on the other side' mentality as a teen. I wished I had straight hair. As an adult I've embraced my curls and wear them proud."

—Nicole Ortega, photographer/writer

Texture: 3b, high-porosity, fine, thick

Regimen: My favorite product regimen is using a styling custard on my towel dried hair, letting it air dry until it's eighty percent dry, diffusing it and then and spraying it with DevaCurl Flexible-Hold hairspray.

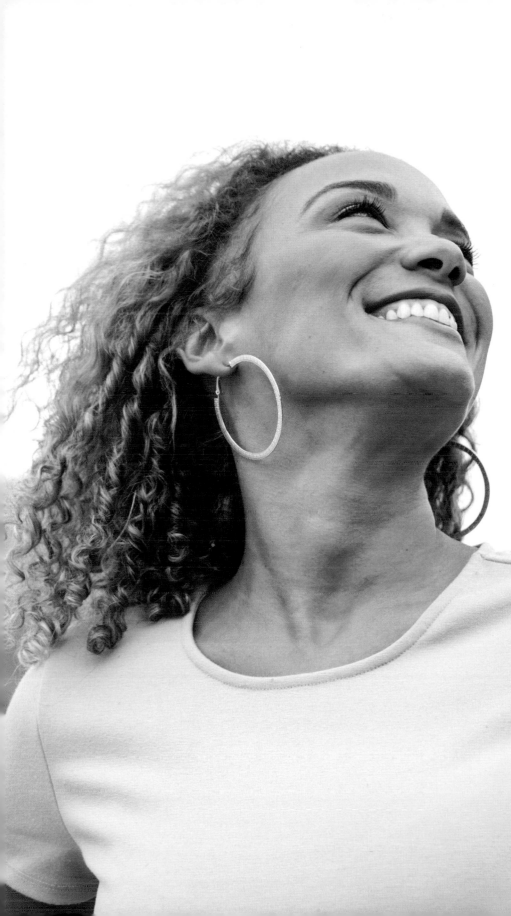

> " I wasn't educated. I didn't know how to style my hair. I didn't embrace it at all or get compliments. When it was curly, it wasn't like people said anything bad. But when I straightened it, I got compliments. There weren't hair products that worked. Now, products help you. I wash, condition, and call it a day."

—Tyesha Vidal, sales distributor of natural hair products

Texture: 3b/3c, low porosity, fine, thick

Regimen: Mixed Chicks Sulfate-Free Shampoo, Mixed Chicks Deep Conditioner, CURLS Blueberry Bliss Leave-in Conditioner and for styling: (wash 'n go) Kinky-Curly Curling Custard (Twist Out) Camille Rose Curl Love (on the 2nd or 3rd day), Design Essentials Coconut Monoi Curl Refresher

knowing and believing that my hair is perfect just the way it is naturally."

In 2011, Isabella Vazquez, who had straightened her hair for most of her life, was chosen to lead the education content team for the launch of Redken's new Curvaceous line for curly hair.

"Do I have to wear my hair curly all the time?" asked Vazquez, editorial hair stylist and founder of the social media channels Curlpopnhair.com and *curlpopworld*.

"That depends on how much you want to affect the market," she was told.

"In that very moment I felt that not only my career would change, but my entire lifestyle would be impacted," says Vazquez. "I set out to live and learn the true life of the curly girl. I would be hanging out with curly girls, talking and understanding what was involved, listening to deep conversations of people who didn't understand and hated their curls. It was then that I made it my mission to impact the industry by exposing salon professionals to what a curly girl *is* and not what a curly girl *should* be from everyone else's point of view. That was the beginning of a journey, and a big deal for me."

This shared journey is why there's such an instant bond between curlies—even total strangers. Gia Lowe recalls walking down the street with her headphones on and seeing a security guard "with her little natural out."

"I felt like I wanted to compliment her hair," says Lowe, a cofounder of Curly Girl Collective (an organization that connects people and brands). "She went right into telling me her story—how long it took her to do her Big Chop (cutting off all her relaxed hair at once), how happy she was to finally wear her hair out. She felt seen. She felt heard. She felt like a part of a community. We were connected at that moment."

The struggle to accept one's curls isn't limited to women.

Therapist and blogger Jor-El Caraballo began his own curly journey in 2009 when he was in graduate school. He was in a program about self-exploration, and it encouraged him to get in touch with a lot of the things affecting his life.

"Hair was a big thing for me," he says.

As a kid growing up in King's Mountain, North Carolina, his hair made him feel out of place. He wore it short and pomaded, sleeping in a wave cap to control his coils.

Away at college in New York City, he decided to grow a big Afro.

"I wanted to express myself differently,"

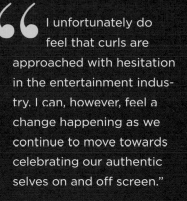

> " I unfortunately do feel that curls are approached with hesitation in the entertainment industry. I can, however, feel a change happening as we continue to move towards celebrating our authentic selves on and off screen."

—Toni Trucks, TV, film, and stage actress

Texture: 3a, high porosity, fine, thin

Regimen: I use Curlisto Botanical Shampoo and Rinse. While my hair is still dripping wet, I detangle with a wide-tooth comb or a wet brush. I then generously apply Curlisto Structure Lotion to lock in my curl shape section by section. I gently shake and scrunch my hair to remove excess moisture as I go. Lastly, I diffuse on low to discourage any frizz.

> "My hair tethers me to a community and culture grounded in heritage, badass-ness and magic. As an individual, my wild and elegant blond, kinky hair has been my most notable physical attribute."

—Michaela Angela Davis, writer, culture critic, and activist

Texture: 4b, high porosity, coarse, thin

Regimen: I use Madam CJ Walker Jamaican Black Castor & Murumuru Oils, Defining Butter Crème, and Madam CJ Walker Scent & Shine Coconut Oil. I'm a grown-ass woman so I use primarily premium products.

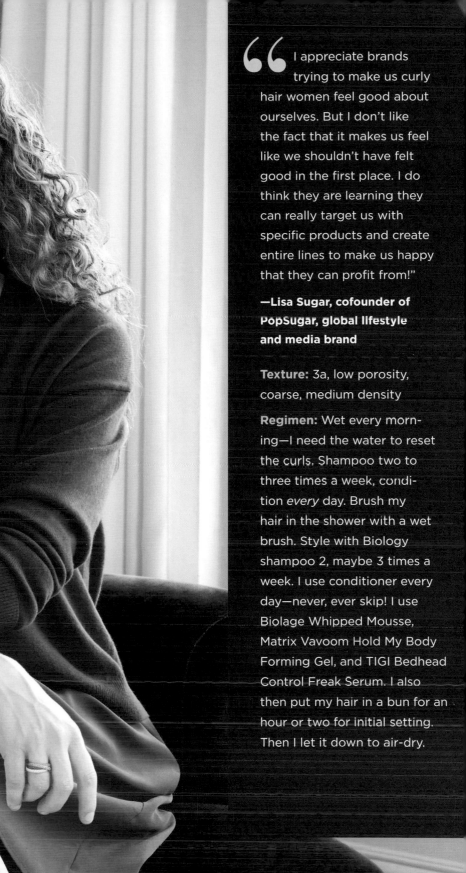

"I appreciate brands trying to make us curly hair women feel good about ourselves. But I don't like the fact that it makes us feel like we shouldn't have felt good in the first place. I do think they are learning they can really target us with specific products and create entire lines to make us happy that they can profit from!"

—**Lisa Sugar, cofounder of PopSugar, global lifestyle and media brand**

Texture: 3a, low porosity, coarse, medium density

Regimen: Wet every morning—I need the water to reset the curls. Shampoo two to three times a week, condition *every* day. Brush my hair in the shower with a wet brush. Style with Biology shampoo 2, maybe 3 times a week. I use conditioner every day—never, ever skip! I use Biolage Whipped Mousse, Matrix Vavoom Hold My Body Forming Gel, and TIGI Bedhead Control Freak Serum. I also then put my hair in a bun for an hour or two for initial setting. Then I let it down to air-dry.

> " My curly hair is an enormous part of my identity—visually, culturally, ethnically. I have not straightened my hair in 10 years."

—Talia Billig, musician, YouTuber

Texture: 3b/3c, high porosity, coarse, very thick

Regimen: I use DevaCurl No-Poo every three days, DevaCurl One Condition on every wash day (every 1 to 2 days), Ultra Defining Gel with a little DevaCurl Set It Free, DevaCurl Styling Cream, and DevaCurl Heaven in Hair Deep Conditioner. I haven't air dried in a long time. I always diffuse

#curl**talk**

We asked NaturallyCurly's Instagram followers when they first felt pretty, having curly hair.

"I was 40 when I finally started using the Curly Girl method and accepted my hair. Love it now and get so many compliments!"

"Just this year I decided to do a big chop and discovered a product that worked great with my hair. No more bad school pictures for me!"

"When I got my first good-enough curly cut, I was shy wearing my curls free for the first time in public. A very cute guy said, 'What perfect hair!' But it still took another three years before I accepted my texture."

"When I got a proper hair cut that matched my curl pattern and face,"

"When my husband (boyfriend at the time) saw me for the first time with my hair out, he was like 'Baby, you so beautiful with your real hair,' and I started my 'transition.'"

"The moment I Big Chopped!"

Caraballo says. "My hair was a manifestation of my growth. For me, it was about being nervous about how people would perceive me."

Like many natural hair influencers, Caraballo's *Mane Man* blog grew out of his own hair experience.

Living curly is a continual process. Sometimes it only takes a bad haircut or a humid day to make you feel like you're right back at square one. Curl acceptance doesn't mean you don't still look in envy at your straight-haired friend who can spend an hour in a sweaty yoga class without a strand moving out of place while your own hair is a frizzy mess.

"I'm still brainwashed by the cultural zeitgeist at that point," says musician and YouTuber Talia Billig, whose curls earned her the nicknamed "Martian" as a child.

She's learning to embrace her hair's unpredictability, and it's now been a decade since she last straightened it.

"I can't predict on any day what it will do. It complements my artistic nature and creativity. It is a very big part of my identity."

NICKNAMES

Kids can be cruel to other kids, latching on with vitriol to any feature that stands out; curly hair is no exception. Cofounder Gretchen Heber's father told her many times that her hair looked like she "combed it with a stick!"

On the following page are a few nicknames endured by members of our community.

And of course there's the perennial "You look like you stuck your finger in a light socket!"

TIPS TO CURL ACCEPTANCE

Find inspiration at NaturallyCurly.com

Get Inspired: Peruse Pinterest, YouTube, Instagram—and of course NaturallyCurly.com—to see all the curly, coily, and wavy styles that are possible.

Knowledge is Power: Education is an important step in loving your curls. That means learning how to take care of your curls, what products and ingredients work best for your hair, and discovering the best techniques for styling your hair. There are numerous sources for this information, including NaturallyCurly.

Connect: Go to any natural hair meet-up and you'll experience the power of curl kinship. There's nothing like a room filled with women rocking their texture to make you

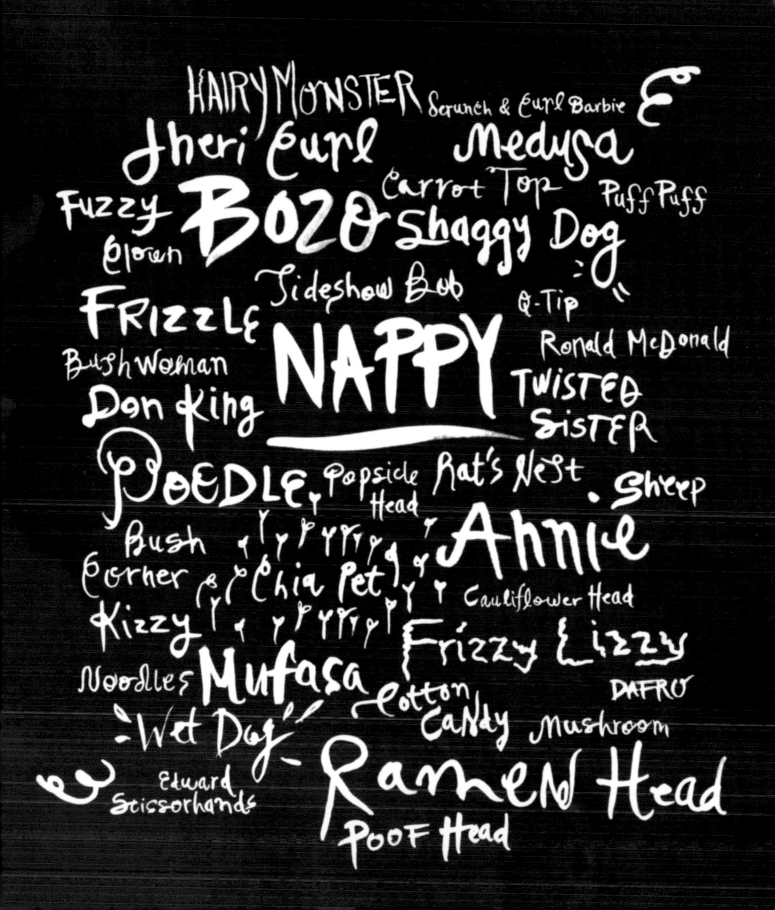

> "I faced a lot of criti-cism in my small town for having hair that wasn't long and straight. Teasing and bullying were a big part of my lack of hair love."

—Alexzandra Jenkins, college student

Texture: 3b/3c, low porosity, coarse, medium density

Regimen: I do the L.O.C. method. My favorite brands are SheaMoisture, It's a 10, and DevaCurl.

feel grateful for your own texture. Or just walk up to a curly on the street and you're likely to forge a friendship over your shared experiences with hair.

Find a Curl Stylist: For so many women with curly and coily hair, getting the right curly cut was life changing. In addition to providing you with a shape that works with your texture and lifestyle, a good stylist can provide priceless styling education.

Tool Time: There are certain tools a curly girl should never be without. Depending on your texture, these critical tools might include a diffuser, a wide-tooth comb, a microfiber towel, or satin pillowcase.

Appreciate: Texture is exotic and unique, with its own personality. It can be your most memorable asset.

"When people describe who I am, they always say the girl with the big curly hair," says award-winning tattoo artist Tiffany Tattooz.

Confidence is Key: If you feel good about your hair, it's contagious. NaturallyCurly published an article in which the writer posted two profiles of herself on Match.com. In one profile, her hair was straight. In the other, it was curly. If her date chose her straight, she showed up curly, and vice versa. She found that if she walked in with her head high and a sense of confidence, the dates went equally well, whether her hair was curly or straight.

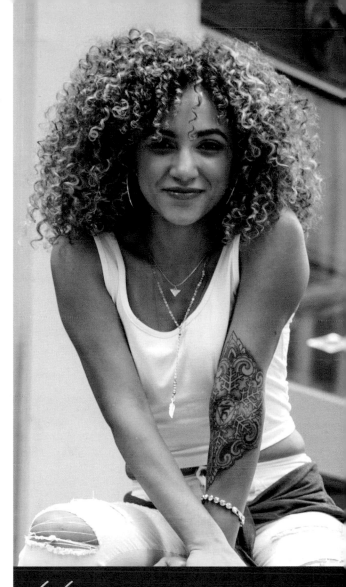

" Five years ago, I transitioned to completely curly hair. When I was in the ugly phase, it made me feel a little insecure. Some people didn't recognize me. They were confused. Now I feel like my curly hair is my signature."

—Tiffany Tattooz, tattoo artist, influencer

Texture: 3c, high porosity, coarse, thick

Regimen: Co-wash with Ouidad Curl Immersion No-Lather Coconut Cream Cleansing Conditioner Co-Wash, condition with Giovanni Direct Leave-in Conditioner, style with DevaCurl Volumizing Foam

> "I think as a young kid, having hair that stood out—literally and figuratively—automatically made me feel like I stood out too. It wasn't that I didn't like it. It just wasn't often that I saw another girl with hair like mine. As I've gotten older, I've found the products and regimen that work for me and realized that I am blessed to have the best of both the hair worlds."

—Jordin Sparks, singer

Texture: 3b/3c, medium-porosity, fine, medium density

Regimen: Pureology Hydrate Shampoo and Conditioner. I leave a little bit of the conditioner in to weigh it down. Then I use half Pureology Nourishing Nectar Styling Gel and half Pureology Color Stylist Illuminating Curl 24-Hour Shaping Lotion. And I let it air dry. I can't use a diffuser or blow dryer because it makes my hair so frizzy!

> My nickname from 6th grade to high school was 'Curly.' It started out bad, but now I own it. People still call me curly, and I'm 30 years old."

—Andrea Barrera, development director for a non-profit

Texture: 3b, high porosity, fine, thick

Regimen: I use DevaCurl No-Poo and DevaCurl Heaven in Hair Intense moisture Treatment every three days. Then I put Style Sexy Not So Hard Up Gel in it. I use silver clips at the roots to get a little volume.

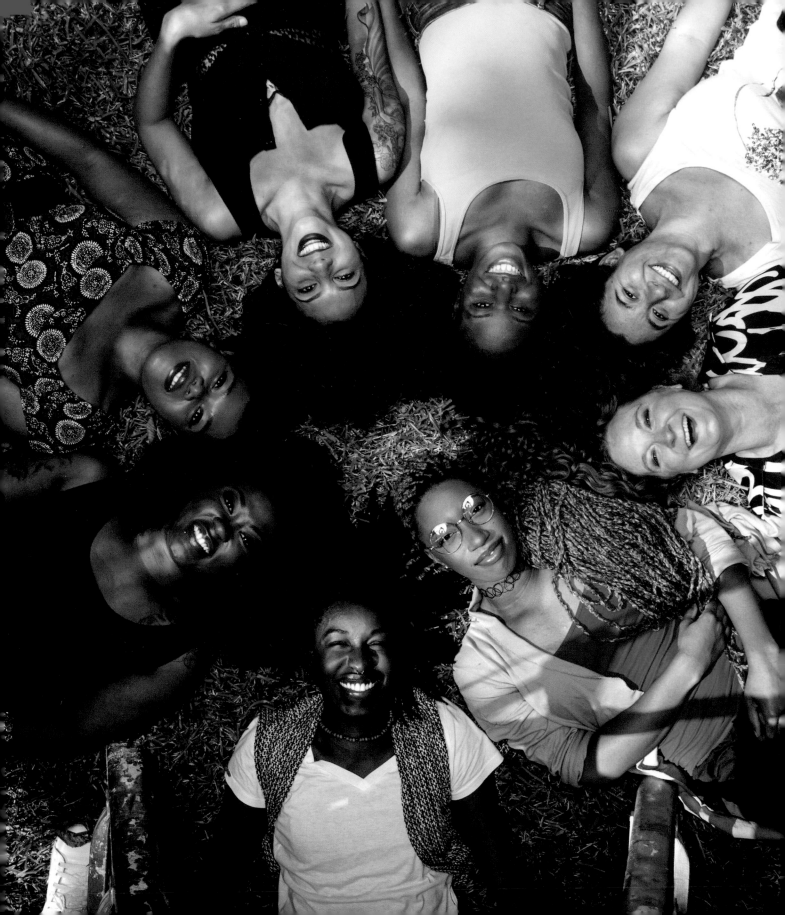

Chapter 3

TEXTURE TYPING—
IT'S MORE THAN JUST CURL PATTERN

Caring for curls can be challenging because so much of the advice —still—is one-size-fits-all. Less-informed sources apply the term "curly" to any non-straight texture, from wavy to super coily and everything in between—a fairly broad and diverse range of hair textures. You may have tried a technique or product not suited to your texture and been discouraged by the results. Or, you may have been given general hair advice based solely on your ethnicity, which may or may not have been appropriate for your specific hair texture or the style you want.

For many years—until the Curl Revolution—the majority of curlies had to figure out their hair care on their own. Even to this day, plenty of misinformation abounds. NaturallyCurly was one of the first online resources to focus on the needs of this under-represented but large group of people—more than 60 percent of the population, by most estimates!

"I *love* sending my potential clients and others to NaturallyCurly.com to learn about their texture, curl type, and more," says stylist and curl expert Scott Musgrave, founder of Curly Hair Artistry, a global network of stylists specializing in curls. "When a client first starts out, they have no clue as to what their hair can potentially do. I want to help them embrace their hair, and texture typing helps with this."

Each head of hair has its own unique characteristics that are defined at the scalp, shaping and influencing the way hair grows and behaves. The more you understand those characteristics—the shape of the follicle, the hair's pattern, and its relationship to moisture—the better.

First, you must learn to identify what type of curl shape and pattern or patterns you have—most curlies have more than one curl texture on their head. When we started NaturallyCurly, we wanted an easy way to take some of the confusion out of caring for hair. We discovered former Oprah Winfrey stylist Andre Walker's hair-typing system—a hair-pattern classification system that uses numbers to identify different levels of curliness, with 1 being straight hair and 4 being super-coily hair. An old approach to curl typing was to lump hair texture into ethnic identities, which didn't account for all the varieties and differences among the curls of women of every race and background. Walker's method made much more sense.

"I didn't want to continue that ethnic myth," said Walker. "I have relatives and friends that are black and their hair types are 1, 2, 3, and 4. I just wanted people to learn what type of hair they have and how to get the best out of it and learn how to take care of it and manage it."

NaturallyCurly adopted Walker's system, adapting it for our readers and focusing on types 2 (wavy) through 4 (coily). The sub classifications, from a to c, are based upon the diameter of the wave, curl or coil. "I'm a 3a because my hair is curly but loose curls."

Although many companies subsequently developed their own curl-typing systems, the system used on NaturallyCurly has become a tool used across the blogosphere—providing a scale that can be used across brands.

Because we addressed a wide range of textures, we attracted and cultivated a diverse community of all ethnicities. It was a system that provided an objective starting point. Often people with completely different ethnic backgrounds share similar curl types.

A person's curl type is only part of the equation. Other factors are equally important in determining which products, cuts, and styling techniques will work best for their hair. Density, thickness, and length are other factors that will influence your curls and will help determine which methods work best for you.

NaturallyCurly's texture-typing system allows curlies to identify curl type, porosity, density, thickness, and length—establishing a complete picture of the nature of your hair and why it does what it does. Armed with

> " I was a young preteen when my waves transformed into curls, and it was pretty hard to swallow at first. All anyone could ever want to be was Jennifer Aniston at that time. NaturallyCurly was HUGE in helping me with my transformation."

—Janell Stephens, founder of Camille Rose Naturals

Texture: 3a/3b, medium porosity, fine, medium density

Favorite Regimen: Once a week I will wash with DevaCurl No-Poo and I love MopTop Daily Conditioner. I use a moisturizing treatment (like Macadamia Professional Nourishing Moisture Masque). I use Curly Hair Solutions Curl Keeper Original daily since I live in south Texas and frequently deal with humidity. I follow up with a cream of some sort, either Curl Junkie Smoothing Lotion or AG Hair Re:coil Curl Activator. On super humid days, I apply Miss Jessie's Jelly Soft Curls gel to help keep my curls springy.

Your hair shaft, or strand, is the part of your hair that you can see. It is primarily made up of two, sometimes three, layers:

- **The Cuticle:** This is the flexible outside layer that covers the hair.

- **The Cortex:** This is the center layer that accounts for the majority of the strand and contains the important lipids, water, and melanin (pigment molecules) that give your hair its color, strength, and elasticity. It's where chemical changes take place when hair is permed, bleached, or relaxed.

- **The Medulla:** Not all strands have a medulla—a middle, innermost layer—it is typically present only in thick, coarse hair. Scientists are still uncertain what the role of the medulla is.

this knowledge, you can customize your search for information, videos, and product recommendations that are most relevant to your unique texture.

Let's get started!

WHAT MAKES HAIR CURLY?

Curly hair is determined by the genes you inherit from your parents, just like the color of your eyes. You probably already know that. But to understand why a curly strand forms, twists, or bends, while a straight strand grows in one direction, you have to look at its root.

Hair is formed below the scalp by keratin protein cells that are pushed up through the skin from the hair bulb. As your hair grows, it moves through a hair follicle, a tube-like pocket that keeps your hair anchored into your skin. The shape of the hair follicle ultimately determines the shape of your strands. A symmetrical follicle produces straight hair. An irregularly shaped follicle creates a curl. (In waves, the follicle is a semi-oval; in coily hair it is a flat-oval shape.) As keratin cells push up through the hair follicle, they receive color from melanin cells and are conditioned by oil from the sebaceous glands, thus affecting the color and porosity of your strands.

To find your texture type, go to NaturallyCurly.com

NATURALLYCURLY'S TEXTURE-TYPING SYSTEM

So how do you find out what your texture type is? Here are few things to keep in mind. First, you must assess your hair in its natural state. What does that entail? Your hair should be properly moisturized and healthy, so you may need to first grow out any heat-damaged hair or chemical treatments before you can evaluate your hair's true shape.

It's also important to keep in mind that most people have a combination of different texture types, so more than one type may apply to you. For example, in terms of curl type, you may be primarily 3c at your crown and front, with some 4a curls in the back. As you go through this guide to learn the components of your particular texture type, use the accompanying information to learn how to care for each section of your hair.

"It's actually uncommon for you to have one texture uniform throughout," says Miko Branch, cofounder of the Miss Jessie's Salon and product line.

You will learn to use this knowledge to bring more consistency to your gorgeous head of curls.

Porosity: Your Hair's Relationship with Moisture

Textured hair is naturally dry, but it's not that simple. To keep your hair soft and conditioned, you must understand your hair's porosity—its ability to absorb and retain moisture. Knowing your porosity is just as important as knowing your curl type, because not all curls handle water, or other moisturizers, the same way. (This is why you probably own a shelf full of partially used bottles of creams and conditioners that did nothing for your curls.)

Porosity varies depending on the condition of your hair cuticle. Remember, the hair cuticle opens and closes to allow moisture in and out of the hair strand. Its ability to do this important job will determine whether your hair's porosity is low, medium, or high.

Low Porosity

When you have low-porosity hair, your cuticle layer is tighter and flatter. Because moisture, oils, and chemical treatments have difficulty penetrating your low-porosity hair, you will need to work extra hard to help it receive moisture. Low-porosity hair benefits from lightweight hydration, so look for water-based

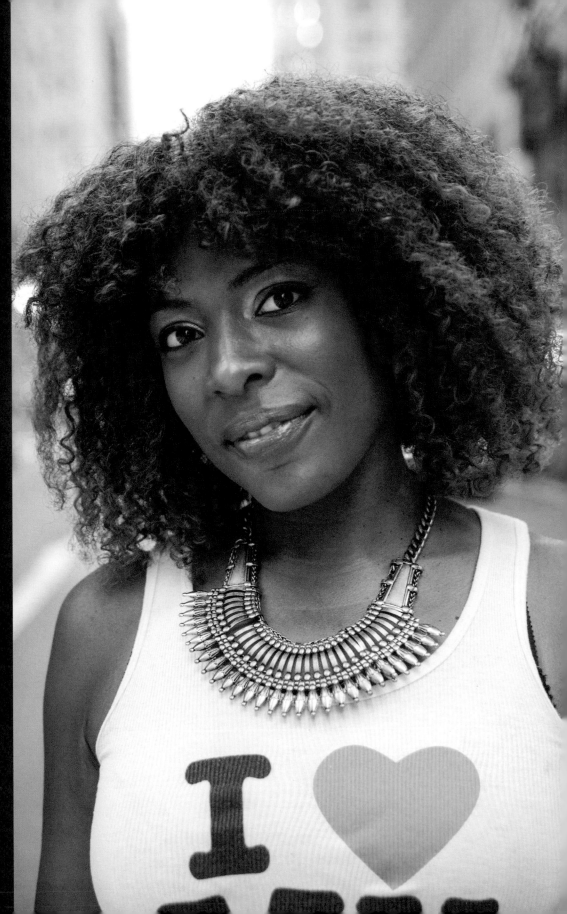

> "When I was 20, I cut all my long, relaxed hair off to a short Afro, and my grandmother hated it. I was the first in my family to go natural. She said 'What did you do?' She looked and talked to me differently. I used to visit her every weekend and we started having confrontations. It taught me that the people closest to you won't always agree with you. But if you stand up for yourself, you never know how you can inspire. Now my mother, aunt, and grandmother are natural."

—Kissa Thompson, founder of Buttafly Unlimited

Texture: 3c/4a, high porosity, coarse, thick

Regimen: Wash with Miss Jessie's Créme de la Créme Conditioning Cream, condition with SheaMoisture Jamaican Black Castor Oil Leave-in Conditioner. I also use coconut and olive oil.

conditioners and hair milks with humectants or non-greasy natural oils with a low molecular weight—like jojoba.

Add heat into your conditioning ritual; a little warm water or a hooded dryer helps lift your cuticle and increase penetration. Steer clear of heavy moisturizers that will sit on your cuticle—making your hair greasy, and avoid protein-based products—they will build up on your hair and make it feel stiff or brittle.

Medium Porosity

Don't feel mediocre if your hair is of medium porosity. Average porosity is a very good characteristic for hair, one in which your cuticle allows the right balance of moisture in and out of your hair. Lucky for you, your curls don't have the same hydration issues as others. Experiment with light- to medium-weight moisturizing conditioners and oils (like pomegranate seed) to keep your curls soft and bouncy. Your hair probably doesn't need protein treatments, so skip them or keep them to a minimum. While your hair probably holds styles and takes processing pretty well, be aware that over time styling and processing can ultimately damage your cuticle and push it into the high-porosity level.

High Porosity

In high-porosity hair, the cuticle layers are both very lifted and farther apart because of texture type or as a result of gaps and holes caused by chemical, mechanical, or environmental damage. Your hair allows too much moisture into the hair, so frizz is always an issue. At the same time, high-porosity hair has the hardest time retaining moisture, so your hair always feels dry or brittle, and strands break more easily. Layer your curls with thicker, heavier leave-in conditioners, creams, and oils to help maintain hydration, and apply protein-rich treatments like aloe and wheat to strengthen the hair shaft.

Hair Density: How Much Hair Do You Have?

Often confused with hair thickness, hair density measures the amount of hair you have on your head, and it affects your hair texture.

Knowing your hair density will help you make smarter choices not only in the styles you wear but the products you use when forming a healthy hair regimen.

To determine density, start with dry hair, because hair that's wet will often look thinner than it really is. Let your hair hang loose in its natural, unparted shape and look at it closely from all different angles. If you can see your scalp very easily, then you have low hair density. If you can see some of your scalp, you have medium hair density. If your scalp is difficult or impossible to see, then you have high hair density.

While it might be difficult to actually increase or decrease the number of hairs that grow out of your head, the appearance of density can be manipulated with products, styling, and the right haircut.

Low Density

Low-density hair will be less than two inches in circumference when the hair is in a ponytail. Volume is always your top concern. You don't have a lot of hair, and can see visible scalp around your crown. You may also have a skimpy ponytail, less than two inches in diameter. Use lightweight products like mousse, dry shampoos, and volumizing shampoos and conditioners with thickening agents to plump up your hair.

Rounded hairstyles, bobs, and blunt cuts can help your hair look fuller.

Medium Density

Your ponytail is two to three inches in circumference when your hair is in a ponytail. The amount of hair you have is manageable. You may see a little scalp. You can play with a variety of products, styles, and cuts. Amp up your volume with a mousse or dry shampoo, or give hair more weight to hang with heavier styling creams or moisturizing butters.

High Density

You have tons of hair and plenty of natural volume—perhaps more than you'd like. No visible scalp shows through and your ponytail is at least four or more inches in circumference. Choose heavy products like gels, creams, butters, and oils to hold curls together and reduce volume. Layered hairstyles help balance volume and remove bulk.

Width: How Thick (and Strong) Are Your Strands?

The width or diameter, also called texture, of your individual strands affects the amount of volume you have, as well as your hair's overall strength, durability, and ability to retain length. Knowing your width will help you realize what your hair can actually handle and what may be getting in the way of your goals. To find your hair width, take a piece of your hair from a brush or comb and hold it up to the light. If the hair is very wide and easily visible, then you have coarse hair. If it's so thin that you can hardly see it, you have fine hair. If your hair appears neither thin nor coarse, you have medium width hair.

Coarse

Your strands may be rough, but they are strong and resistant to damage. Because they are more robust, your hair easily handles heat, styling wear and tear, and processing, so you can experiment with many different styles and treatments. Use rich moisturizers, butters, and oils to help keep your thicker strands soft and smooth.

Medium

Your hair width falls somewhere between coarse and fine, strong and elastic, and has a fair amount of volume. In many ways your hair is low maintenance—it's relatively easy to grow out your hair as long as you don't overdo the hot tools and processing. Creams and butters will help to control your curls, while volumizers can give you extra body when you want it.

Fine

Your hair is the thinnest and most delicate of all the hair textures, but you can add extra bulk with volumizing stylers and thickening shampoos and conditioners. The reason your hair takes forever to grow or won't reach past a certain length is because it's the most vulnerable to damage and breaking. Avoid heat and use low-manipulation hairstyles to prevent breakage and keep your strands healthy. Depending on your density, volume may or may not be an issue for you.

Length: Why Do Curls Take So Long to Grow?

All hair grows an average of six inches a year—whether you are straight or curly. It can be a little more or less depending on your health, nutrition, stress levels, and hormones. However, for curlies with tighter curl patterns, it can take much longer to see any gains in length because your growth appears horizontally rather than vertically due to your curl's shrinkage or spring factor. Curly strands also tend to be delicate, which makes breakage another problem. As you've learned, factors like porosity and width affect how well your hair can withstand damage and breakage. So it can take a lot of extra work to keep your curls healthy enough to gain precious inches. If you want long hair, you'll need to consider everything from conditioning, to gentle detangling and styling, to avoiding chemicals and heat, to getting regular trims. The shorter your hair, the less you have to maintain. You'll also have more freedom with your style because you can just cut away the damage. The beauty of your curls is that they change and evolve as they grow—so learn to embrace them at every length.

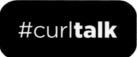

HOW HAS YOUR TEXTURE CHANGED OVER YOUR LIFE?

A child with silky fine hair may end up with a head full of kinky curls when puberty hits. Another baby may start out with fine ringlets only to have them turn stick straight when she gets older.

Throughout life, we see changes in our hair textures. In fact, hair texture technically changes every five to seven years.

The hair of a newborn is very soft and very fine. The diameter of the hair thickens as we enter childhood or early adolescence. As we move into adulthood and then older, the hair again changes, becoming finer again in our forties and fifties. Some of these changes are inevitable, destined by genetics or natural hormone changes; others are influenced by environmental factors or medications.

We asked our community members how their hair has changed over their lives:

"I looked like Annie (minus the red) as soon as it started growing. Now at 40 it's straightening. I learned to love it early on, and now I'm frustrated at the change."

"Wavy from birth, full blown curls during puberty!"

"I've been seriously ill since my twenties, but now that I recovered, my hair is full of life again and so am I! It is the biggest gift!"

"I was 24 when I got acne, wisdom teeth, grew an inch, and got curly hair."

"My coils got tighter while I was pregnant."

"My hair was super thick and curly when I was younger. Then, I dyed it a lot and straightened, so my curls died completely. After my Big Chop, it came back thick and healthy."

"I started out straight, then got wavy after puberty. Still wavy now but it pretty much transforms into a ball of frizz."

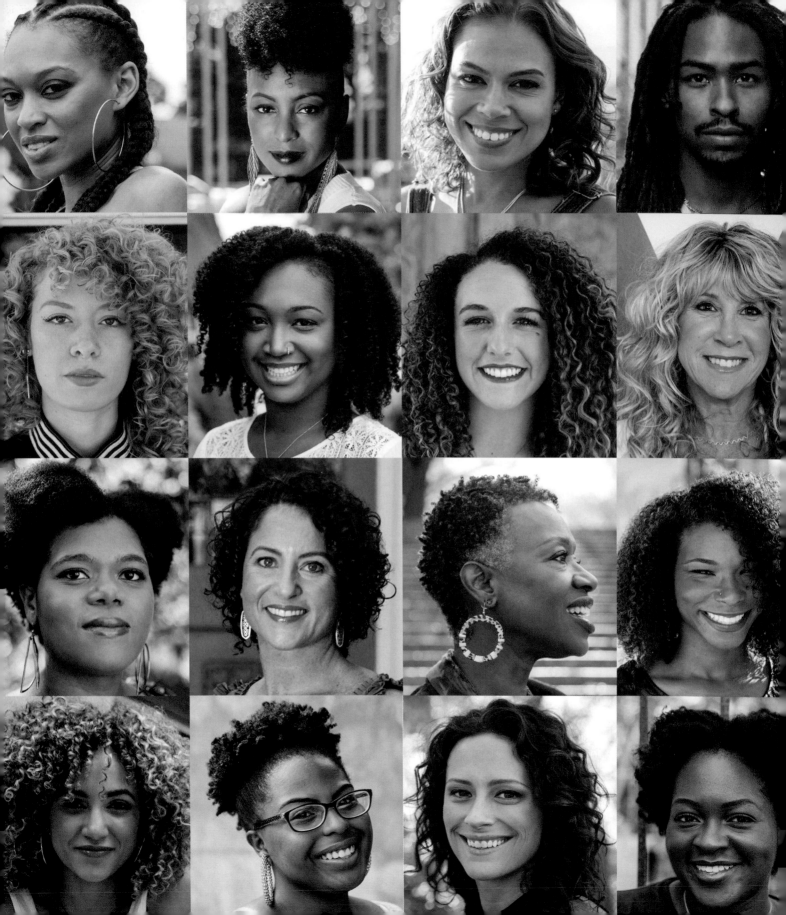

CURL PATTERN GUIDE: WHAT'S YOUR TYPE?

Check out our descriptions below. Remember that determining your curl pattern is a starting point to finding the right products and cuts for your hair. If you need more guidance, go to NaturallyCurly.com.

TYPE 2: WAVY HAIR

Type 2 texture is not quite straight and not completely curly, with the spectrum of hair ranging from loose loops to coarse, thick S-shaped waves combined with curls. Type 2 texture is typically flatter at the root and lays close to the head, getting curlier from the ears down. Waves can get frizzy and limp, so finding the right moisturizers and products that deliver hold are top concerns.

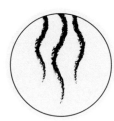

Type 2a

Your waves are fine and thin, with a loose, tousled texture. Their lack of volume and definition means that products can weigh them down easily and strands can become straight.

YOUR CELEB CURL SISTERS: NATALIE DORMER, VANESSA HUDGENS, AND ARIZONA MUSE

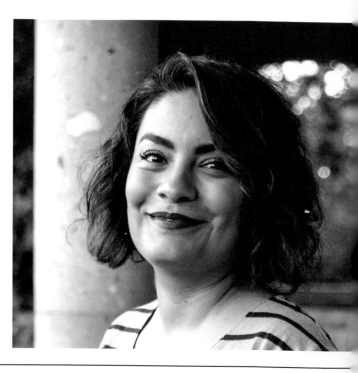

" Before I had a pixie, I had really long hair. Once I cut it, the texture came out. Some days I have ringlets. I'm having so much fun with it. I'm only 5' 1" so I like adding height to my hair. It draws attention and I do love that."

—Leticia Leal, preschool teacher, children's cooking instructor, lead singer in a Van Halen and a Devo cover band

Texture: 2a, medium porosity, medium width, medium density

Regimen: I use OGX Moroccan Quenching Coconut Curls Shampoo, Conditioner, and Curling Styling Milk.

> "When I was young in Lubbock, where it's super dry, my hair was super straight. I even got my hair permed. Then I got a short pixie when I was 13. I loved it short, but there were a lot of mean kids who teased me, so I let it start growing. I moved to Austin and went through puberty and my hair grew in a totally different texture."

—Carley Deardoff, college student and executive assistant

Texture: 2a, low porosity, fine, thick

Regimen: I use Kenra Professional Curl Co-Wash, Kenra Professional Curl Styling Conditioner and some coconut oil.

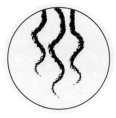

Type 2b

Your hair is mostly straight at the roots and falls into more defined S-shaped waves from the mid-lengths to the ends. It is a medium texture with some frizz at the crown.

YOUR CELEB CURL SISTERS: BETHANY COSENTINO, CHARLI XCX, JASMINE V, JESSICA CHASTAIN, AND ALY MICHALKA

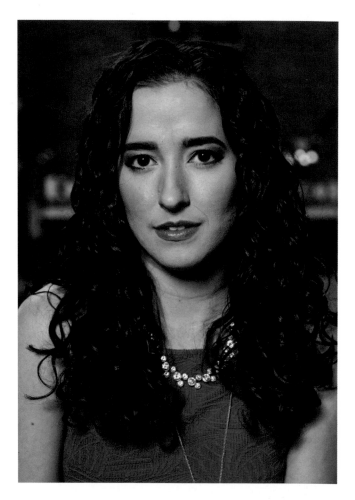

"My mom had super curly hair in the '70s, and felt very tortured by the trend of long, straight blonde hair. She talks about her hair almost like a trauma. As a mom, she celebrated our curls. She sent such a strong message about how we don't need to straighten our hair for events. I didn't realize that curly hair was an emotional issue."

—Jessica Kahkoska, podcast host

Texture: 2b, high porosity, fine, medium

Regimen: I use Shea Moisture Coconut and Hibiscus Curl and Shine conditioner and Kinky Curly custard.

> "I went through a bit of a crisis when I had a bleach disaster. My hair was breaking off—it was traumatic and terrible. I hid inside a little while. My thickness is finally back. I can feel my curl again. Even though it was terrible, the bleach accident was a blessing in disguise. Now that my natural color is growing in, I realize color was affecting my curl pattern."

—Diane Mary Montalto, wavy influencer and founder of Dianemary126 social media platform

Texture: 2b, high porosity, fine, thick

Regimen: I use the Raw Curls Organics line, Wavy Swavy Cleanser and Conditioner, the Ouidad Curl Immersion line, and Ouidad Mongongo Oil.

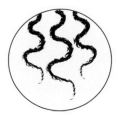

Type 2c

Your waves are more defined and start at the roots, then mix with curls and ringlets. This texture is typically thick or coarse, and prone to frizzing.

YOUR CELEB CURL SISTERS: SALMA HAYEK, TAYLOR SWIFT, YASMIN SEWELL, MAGGIE GYLLENHAAL, AND ADRIENNE BAILON

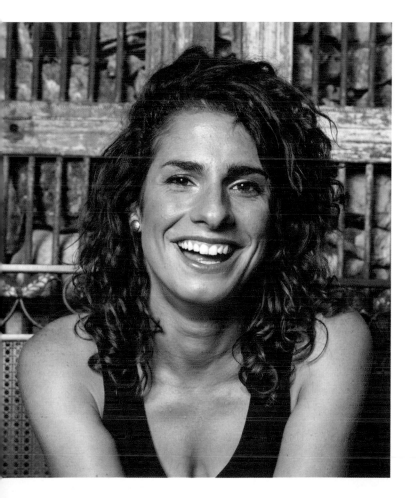

66 In high school, I tried to straighten it. Then I said 'Screw that!' Now, I totally embrace it. I can't remember the last time I saw my hair straight. If I need it to be straight for a role, I wear a wig."

—Rachel Pallante, actor, singer, comedian

Texture: 2c/3a, high porosity, fine, medium density

Regimen: Water, Herbal Essences Totally Twisted Curl Boosting Mousse or Curly Sexy Hair Curl Power Spray Foam Curl Enhancer

TYPE 3: CURLY HAIR

Type 3s range from lightly curly to tight, curly tendrils, and usually have a combination of textures. They are defined and springy with more height and volume at the root than type 2s. Curly hair may appear coarse because it has so much natural body, but its texture is actually soft and fine.

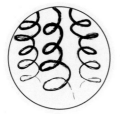

Type 3a

You have big, loose curls and spirals similar in circumference to a piece of thick sidewalk chalk. Your curls tend to be shiny with a well-defined S-shape. Blow-outs are usually no problem for you, nor is styling your hair in its natural state.

> **YOUR CELEB CURL SISTERS: LORDE, ANNALYNNE MCCORD, AND KIMBERLY PERRY**

" I used to hate my hair curly. Now I feel free. When I wear my hair straight now, I feel like 'I need my curls back.'"

—Crystal Collazo, stylist and curly influencer

Texture: 3a/3b, high porosity, fine, thick

Regimen: DevaCurl Light Defining Gel and DevaCurl One Condition

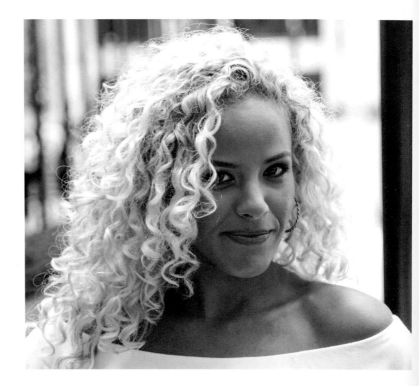

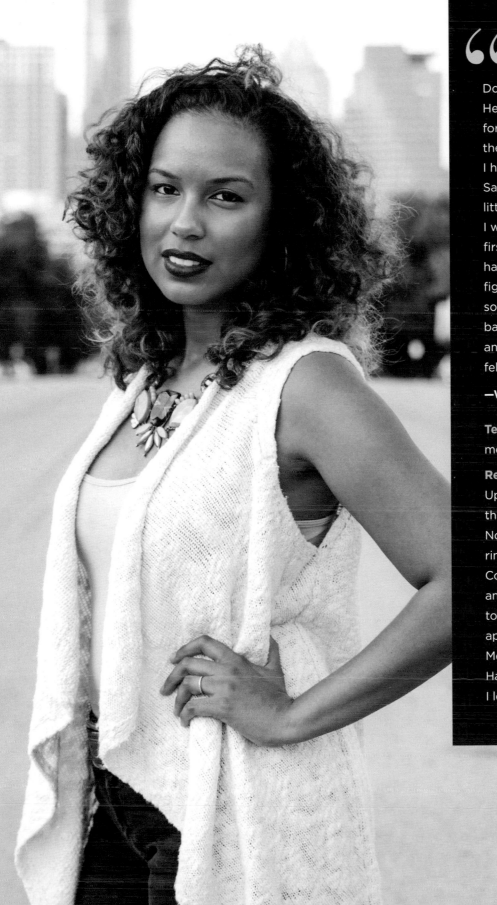

> "My parents were born in the Dominican Republic, and Dominicans in my Washington Heights neighborhood are well known for their talented hair stylists and the magical "Dominican Blowouts"! I had been getting a blowout every Saturday morning since I was very little. When I was around 11 years old, I washed my hair on my own for the first time ever. Although I knew my hair was curly by this age, I had to figure out what to do with it! I found some pink Queen Helene gel in the bathroom cabinet and put it all over and my hair came out so BOMB!! I fell in love!"

—Walki Raposo, social worker

Texture: 3a, low porosity, fine, medium density

Regimen: I use Alba Botanica Drink It Up Hawaiian Coconut Milk Shampoo and then I apply Macadamia Professional Nourishing Moisture Masque. After rinsing that out, I condition with As I Am Coconut CoWash Cleansing Conditioner and rinse with cold water. I use a T-shirt to squeeze a little water out and then apply Proclaim Shea Butter Leave-in Moisturizer and put in Carol's Daughter Hair Milk Alcohol-Free Styling Gel. Then, I let my hair dry naturally.

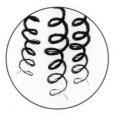

Type 3b

Your springy curls can vary from ringlets to corkscrews. They are voluminous and have a circumference similar to a Sharpie marker. Type 3b hair lacks the shine of 3a curls and tends to be coarse and dense, and may experience some shrinkage as it dries.

YOUR CELEB CURL SISTERS: ANNA SHAFFER, JULIANNA MARGULIES, TAE HECKARD, AND JASMINE SANDERS

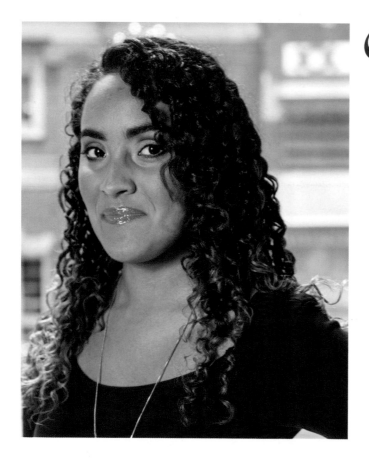

" I'm Dominican, and in my culture, people don't realize how beautiful curls are. My mom and both sisters still straighten, and I'm trying to get them to let their hair go curly. I like my curls better than straightening."

—Elizabeth Almonte, group leader for an after-school program

Texture: 3b, low porosity, fine, thin

Regimen: I use an olive oil pre-'poo treatment a half hour before washing. Then vinegar or SheaMoisture Yucca & Plantain Anti-Breakage Strengthening Shampoo, Superfruit Multi-Vitamin Hair Masque, Kinky Curly Knot-Today Leave-In Conditioner and Sheamoisture. Finally, Coconut & Hibiscus Curl Enhancing on the ends.

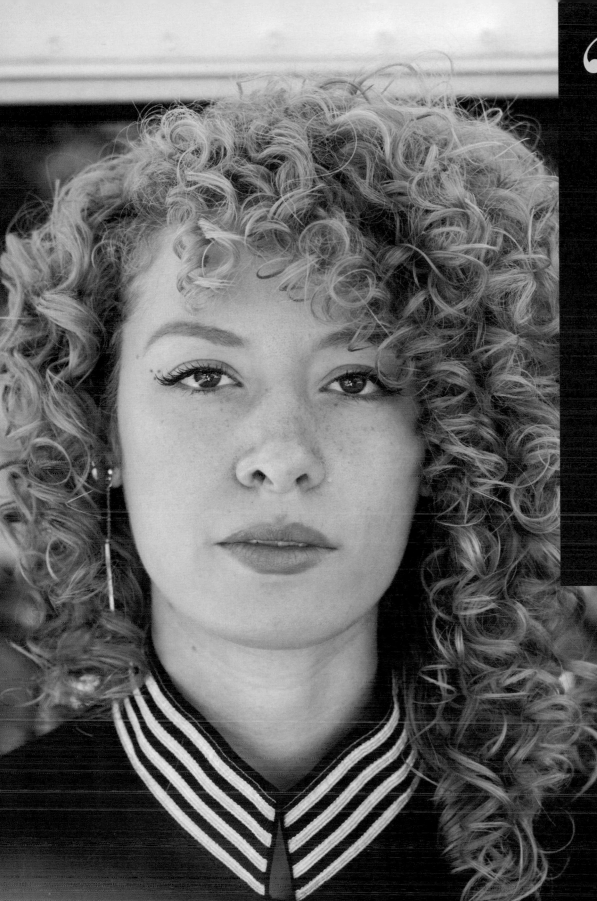

> "It's been curly since high school. I used to straighten it twice a year. I stopped doing that a few years ago. I don't care to. I feel like I look weird with straight hair. It makes me look older."

—Ayshia Collier, founder of Curly Crown, a hair tool that creates volume

Texture: 3b, low porosity, fine, thin

Regimen: I don't shampoo any more. I co-wash with DevaCurl One Condition. Then I use my fingers to distribute Kinky-Curly Knot Today Leave-in Conditioner spray and Oyin Handmade Fruits & Berries.

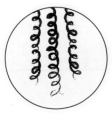

Type 3c

You have very dense, tightly packed corkscrews that are the circumference of a pencil or a straw, usually with a combination of both curly and coily textures. Type 3c tends to experience the most volume but also the most shrinkage of curls.

> **YOUR CELEB CURL SISTERS: TRACEE ELLIS ROSS, LEELA JAMES, TESSA THOMPSON, JURNEE SMOLLET BELL, AND KELIS**

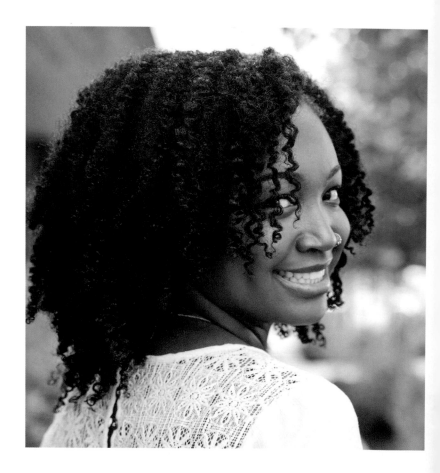

"I've been natural for two years. I wouldn't trade my hair for anything. When I do braid my hair, it looks like the waves you see at the beach and that is AWESOME!"

—Ashley Johnson, event planner

Texture: 3c/4a, low porosity, coarse, thick

Regimen: I just spray some water, put on some Cantu Shea Butter Leave-in Conditioner, and pull my hair into a crown.

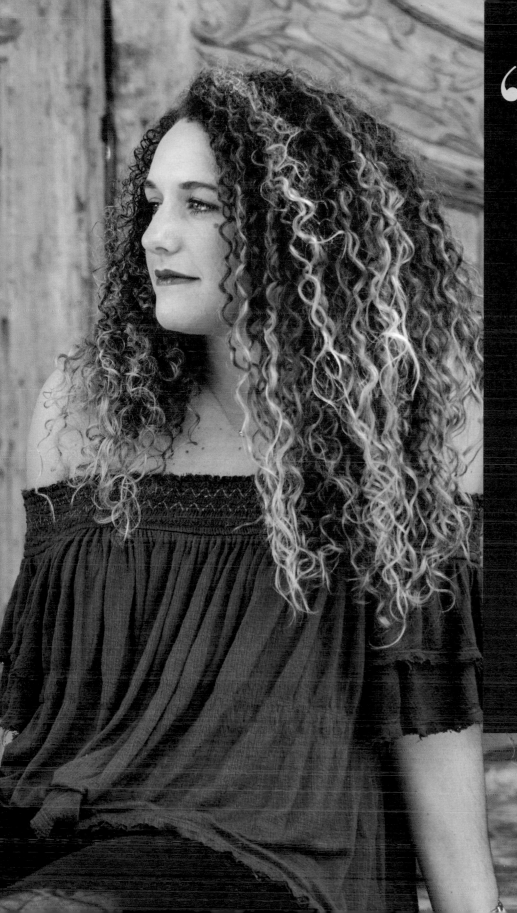

> " I noticed it's such a unique part of me. People notice it a lot more. For some reason, I'll be at a restaurant or out and about, and multiple people will compliment me on my hair. And I'll be like, 'Thanks!' That makes me feel good."

—Morgan Marshall, physical therapist

Texture: 3b/3c, high porosity, coarse, thick

Regimen: I rinse with Pureology Hydrate Conditioner, every day, running my fingers through it. I put Moroccan Oil Treatment throughout my hair and apply Aunt Jackie's Don't Shrink Flaxseed Elongating Curling Gel in one side at a time. I then flip over and scrunch my hair with a microfiber glove and put Kenra Volume Mousse in and scrunch again with the microfiber glove all while flipped upside down. After that, I use a diffuser to completely dry my hair. Once it's dry, I put more Moroccan oil Treatment in and spritz with a little hairspray.

TYPE 4: COILY HAIR

Type 4 hair is fine and thin or wiry and coarse, with densely packed coils. Coily hair may seem robust, but it's actually the most fragile hair texture, because it has the fewest cuticle layers to protect it from dryness. Type 4 hair is more prone to damage and breakage from heat styling and chemical treatments. Its top concerns are maintaining moisture, avoiding tangles, and counteracting shrinkage.

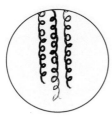

Type 4a

Your dense, springy coils are either wiry or fine and have the circumference of a crochet needle. They are tightly coiled, experience a lot of shrinkage, and have a visible S-pattern.

YOUR CELEB CURL SISTERS: TEYONNAH PARIS, ANDREA LEWIS, YAYA DACOSTA, AND SOPHIE OKONEDO

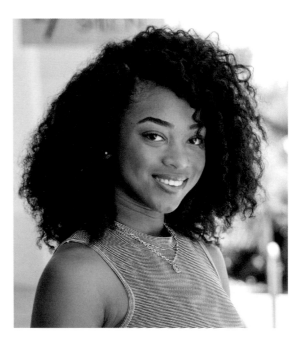

" As a sophomore, I'd seen a lot of pictures of people with curly hair and I thought I might give it a try. On the first day, I was nervous about what people would say. When I got a lot of compliments, I started thinking I should do it more. It helps me stand out."

—Tierra LeYanna, high school student

Texture: 4a, high porosity, coarse, thick

Regimen: Every three days, I use Infusium 23 Moisture Replenishing Shampoo, Cantu Shea Butter Leave-in Conditioning Repair Cream and Cantu Coconut Curling Cream. I twist it over night and then untwist it in the morning.

> "I am not my hair, but my hair is totally an essential part of me. It's my crowning glory, but it's also not something I'm super precious about. I've learned that hair is just hair, and it definitely grows back, so I always try to have fun with it!"

—Cassidy Blackwell, senior manager brand marketing, founder of NaturalSelection blog

Texture: 4a, medium porosity, fine, thick

Regimen: Wash 'n go! The simpler, the better. I like to let my hair, which is named Lola, be free!

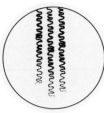

Type 4b

Instead of curling or coiling, your hair bends in sharp angles like the letter Z. The curl is tighter and less defined—about the circumference of a pen—with strands that range from fine and thin to wiry and coarse. 4b coils are densely packed and experience about 75 percent shrinkage.

YOUR CELEB CURL SISTERS: CHRISETTE MICHELE, SOLANGE KNOWLES, JADE COLE, WILLOW SMITH, AND SYESHA MERCADO

" I didn't know anyone in my family who was natural. It was a foreign concept. Lauryn Hill was my inspiration. I was in love with her. I noticed that she was natural and I started to question if I could ever wear my hair natural."

—Natasha Gaspard, founder and executive producer of Mane Moves Media

Texture: 4b, high porosity, fine, thick

Regimen: Creme of Nature Argan Oil Leave-in Conditioner, Cream of Nature Argan Pudding Perfection, SheaMoisture Coconut & Hibiscus Curl Enhancing Smoothie and SheaMoisture African Black Soap Purification Masque.

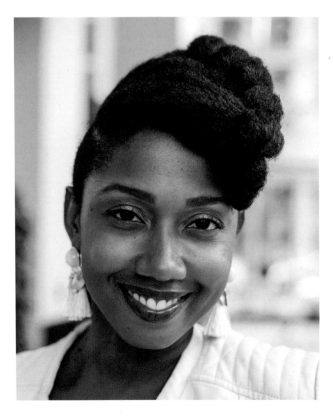

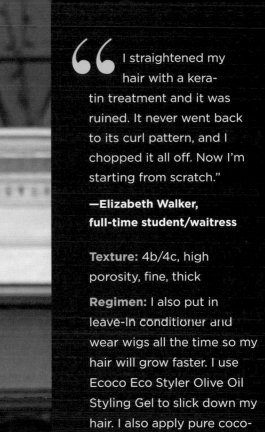

> "I straightened my hair with a keratin treatment and it was ruined. It never went back to its curl pattern, and I chopped it all off. Now I'm starting from scratch."

—Elizabeth Walker, full-time student/waitress

Texture: 4b/4c, high porosity, fine, thick

Regimen: I also put in leave-in conditioner and wear wigs all the time so my hair will grow faster. I use Ecoco Eco Styler Olive Oil Styling Gel to slick down my hair. I also apply pure coconut oil as a moisturizer.

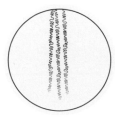

Type 4c

Your densely packed hair is similar to a 4b, but experiences less definition and more shrinkage—75 percent or more. The tightly coiled strand texture ranges from super fine, thin, and soft to wiry and coarse and is very delicate.

YOUR CELEB CURL SISTERS: LUPITA NYONG'O, VIOLA DAVIS, INDIA ARIE, ERYKAH BADU, AND AJUMA NASENYANA

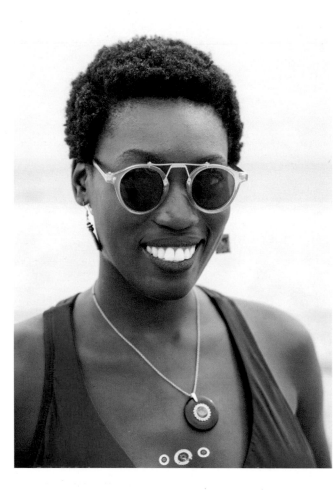

" I never really knew my texture. I woke up one morning and realized that I'm a 30-year-old woman who has never seen her true curl pattern. But I'm so much happier. I like that I'm not trying to be anything other than myself."

—Julia Kwamya, actor and songwriter/music producer

Texture Type: 4c, low porosity, coarse, super thick

Regimen: I use Shea butter and products from Carol's Daughter, DevaCurl, and Viviscal.

> ❝ I had never seen my hair natural. I thought 'It's a part of me I don't know what it looks like.' I figured I could relax it if I didn't like it. I love it!."

—Alaina Flannigan, PhD student in educational psychology

Texture: 4c, high porosity, coarse, thick

Regimen: I use SheaMoisture Manuka Honey & Mafura Oil Intensive hydration shampoo and conditioner twice a week, mixture of Kinky-Curly Knot Today Leave-in conditioner with tea tree oil, distilled water, and aloe vera juice.

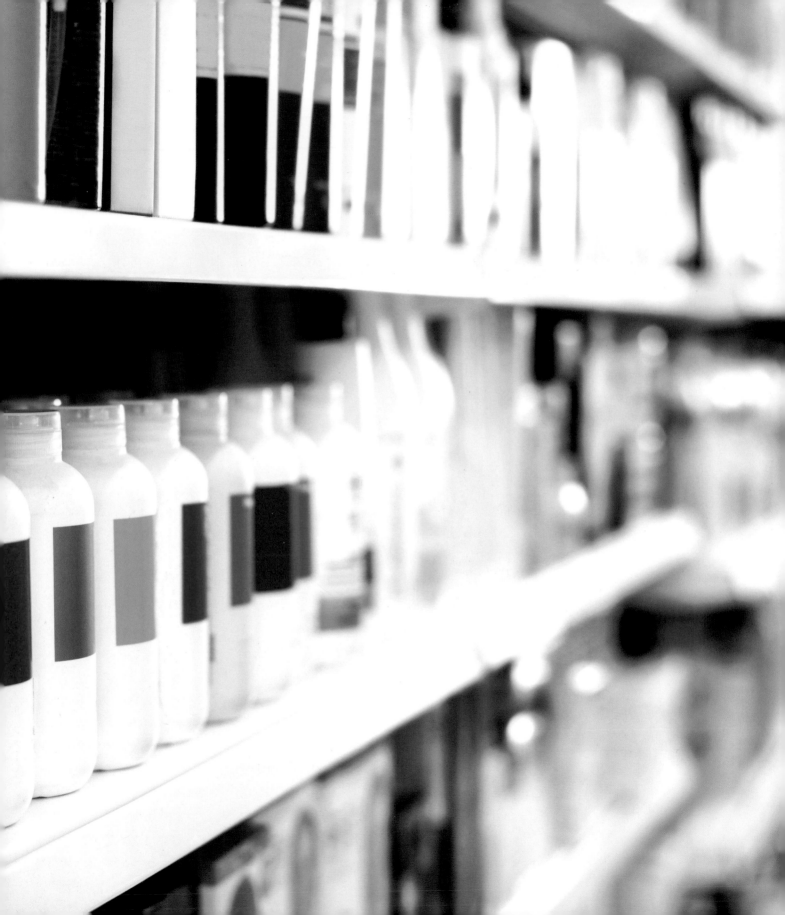

Chapter 4

CREATING YOUR CURLY REGIMEN—

WHAT PRODUCTS TO USE & WHEN

Maria Santos just started her curly journey and is trying to find the right routine for her 3b curls. This means trying a lot of products—her cabinet is filled with nearly three-dozen bottles and tubes. She has so many hair products that her partner has said, "No more products in this house until you're done with these. We don't have the room!"

Healthy curls and coils don't happen by accident. It takes the right routine along with the right combination of products to achieve your ideal texture. For nearly two decades, NaturallyCurly has helped thousands of curlies figure out how to perfect a curl routine—from how, when, and with what products to use to cleanse and condition, to the best products to layer together.

You will notice that nearly every curly featured in this book has a different

regimen—different combinations of products from over a hundred different brands. Most of them say they regularly tweak their routine depending on the weather, their style, or the condition of their hair.

To ensure that your hair gets the care it needs, it's good to create at least a basic regimen that includes cleansing, conditioning, and deep conditioning.

"Hair likes to be on a regimen," says celebrity natural hairstylist Felicia

Leatherwood. "It ensures that you schedule regular time for your curls, which produces better, more consistent results."

For a newcomer to the curly world, figuring out what to use can seem a little overwhelming. One of the most amazing effects of the Curl Revolution is the multitude of new products now available. In fact, entire product categories have sprung up that never existed before, including many created by curlies themselves.

Before the Curl Revolution began, you simply bought shampoo. Now, however, the array of cleansing products is dizzying— no-'poos, pre-'poos, cleansing conditioners, clarifying cleansers, moisturizing shampoos, and co-washes. Conditioners? You can choose from leave-in conditioners, daily conditioners, detanglers, moisturizers, deep conditioners, and dry conditioners. To further complicate things, the lines between cleansers and conditioners have blurred in some cases.

Also overwhelming is the vast array of styling products developed especially for curls and coils—gels, mousses, creams, puddings, milks, custards, pomades, and more.

"The most significant change in the natural hair industry is the varying product options that are being offered," says stylist and educator Diane Bailey, who started working with texture four decades ago. "When I started caring for natural hair exclusively, there were very few products offered to nurture our hair and scalp. I made my own 'kitchen solutions' for textured hair. Currently the influx of natural products—in combination with the rise of social media and the inspiration from the enthusiastic influencers—has pushed the natural hair industry into the mainstream."

Product selection should vary by texture type, the condition of the hair, your lifestyle, and your hairstyle.

"It all depends on the head," says Ana Paula Cota, a senior stylist at Devachan Salon in New York City. "You should personalize your products according to your hair texture and your desired outcome."

> **"I'm the girl who went to the hair salon every week to relax my hair. My family didn't really embrace the texture. The first month I let it curl. I looked in the mirror and felt ugly. Now I love it."**
>
> **—MARIA SANTOS, MEDICAL ASSISTANT**

"I hated my hair for many years because I wasn't given the proper training and tools to manage it. I now love it!!! I get so many compliments. It's amazing what the right products can do for curly hair!"

—Kennett Nicole Pyles, restaurant manager

Texture: 3a, medium porosity, coarse, thick

Regimen: I use Suave The Keratin for Smooth Hair, Herbal Essences Totally Twisted Silkening Detangler, followed by a tiny bit of Herbal Essences Totally Twisted Curl Boosting Mousse. Then I use Tigi Catwalk Curls Rock amplifier, toss my hair a bit, and go.

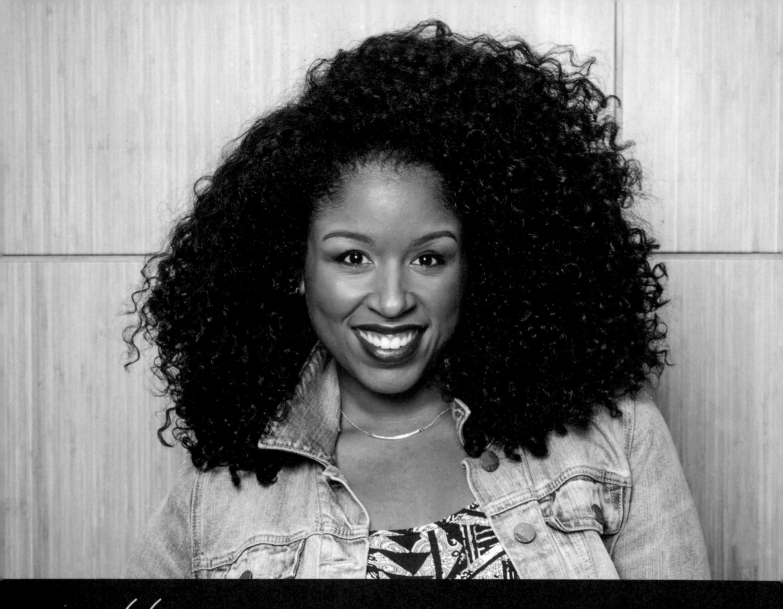

"People still have a lot of issues with selecting products. There's so much conflicting information that they can't see the difference between a good product and good product marketing. Don't throw your common sense out the window when it comes to your hair. You'll find what you like. You don't have to use everything."

—Monica Stevens, hair stylist and blogger MoKnowsHair

Texture: 3b-ish, medium porosity, fine, thick

Regimen: (Wash 'n go) Softsheen Carson Hydrasteam Shampoo, Aveda Damage Remedy Moisturizing Shampoo and Mask (once or twice a month), Ouidad Ultra-Nourishing Cleansing Oil and Ouidad Melt Down Extreme Repair Mask (every 4–6 weeks), Softsheen Carson Hydra Steam Moisturizing System Sulfate-Free Cleanser and mask (most often, weekly with a steamer). I also use Mixed Chicks Leave-in Conditioner as a styler, with CHI Deep Brilliance Silk Reflection reflect, and diffuse with a FHI salon pro-2000-dryer.

For example, you might choose different products if you're going to work versus if you're going to a fancy dinner party. If you have fine, wavy hair, you will need to find products that aren't too heavy. Coilies, on the other hand, may need a thicker product with more moisture.

And then, of course, all this careful product selection is often thrown into disarray the minute the weather changes. What works one season—or one day—may not work the next, depending on heat and humidity.

Being a curly means an ongoing process of discovery, which is why many members of our community proudly call themselves "product junkies." We're not "one shampoo and one conditioner" type of people. Our showers and cabinets are usually filled with dozens of products.

Our favorite Instagrammer may post a photo on Tuesday showing her mane when using a curl cream from a new brand, and, lo and behold, on Wednesday there's a line of curlies at the store wanting to purchase it.

NaturallyCurly wants to make it easier for you to find the routines and product or products that work for you.

CLEANSING: TO 'POO OR NOT TO 'POO

Jessica Kahkoska's hair turned curly when she hit puberty. "My mom (a curly who has been a NaturallyCurly member since 2002) said 'You're going to stop shampooing,'" she says.

Washing one's hair seems like a straightforward step in a person's hair routine. But, it's actually one of the most controversial topics in the curly community. Volumes have been written about what the best techniques and products are for cleansing curls, what ingredients should and should not be in your products, or if you should cleanse at all.

What we've learned—from both experts and community members—is that there is no one right answer. There are some general guidelines that can help you determine how often you cleanse and what product you use to wash your hair. The proper cleansing regimen can have a huge impact, affecting not only the appearance of your curls but also the overall health of your hair and scalp.

In the curly world, 'poo refers not only to shampoo, but also to the types of ingredients in the formula. Traditional shampoos contain cleansing detergents called sulfates that are designed to remove oils, dirt, dead skin, and styling product residue, and to help the formula lather.

However, sulfates can be harsh on both your hair—stripping moisture—and your scalp—causing irritation. Many curl experts warn against using anything that suds or lathers, and recommend instead using mild cleansing formulas (labeled sulfate-free or low-'poo). People who eschew shampoos with sulfates (and therefore also shun products that require sulfates to remove them) are said to be following a "no-'poo routine."

The term "squeaky clean" has become a nonstarter for many in the curly world. Though we all want our hair to be clean, we don't want to strip our hair of the necessary oils it needs to stay healthy.

Some curlies use cleansing creams (called co-washes, cleansing conditioners, and no-'poo) to avoid stripping natural oils from curls. Other curlies actually cleanse with their conditioner, which is where "co-wash" got its name.

An early, prominent proponent of the no-'poo concept was Lorraine Massey, founder of the Devachan Salon in New York and author of *Curly Girl: The Handbook*, a book that quickly became a hair care bible for many curly girls. Combined with Devachan's DevaCurl line of hair care products, the *Curly Girl* book proposed a new routine (sometimes referred to as the CG method) that eliminates the use of sulfates and silicones. Now many stylists and brands have embraced different versions of this routine.

"I believe you should use co-washes or cleansing conditioners as often as possible, because you should retain as much moisture as you can for curly hair," says Lisa Price, creator of the Carol's Daughter hair care line.

Of course there are exceptions to these guidelines. A clarifying cleanse with a "stripping/clarifying" shampoo may be beneficial and occasionally necessary for co-washers to remove product buildup and debris to keep their hair and scalps healthy. If a favorite product has stopped working, the culprit could be product buildup. If a commercial clarifying shampoo isn't to your liking, try a natural alternative, such as a rinse made with apple cider vinegar or baking soda.

Whichever clarifying method you choose, the key is to do it infrequently, and only as necessary.

Price says she co-washes once a week and shampoos every three weeks. "There are times I feel like I need to have lather. It's just that I don't think that we need it quite as often as we think we do."

So—back to regular cleansing: How often do you need to cleanse your curls? Well, the answer ultimately depends on

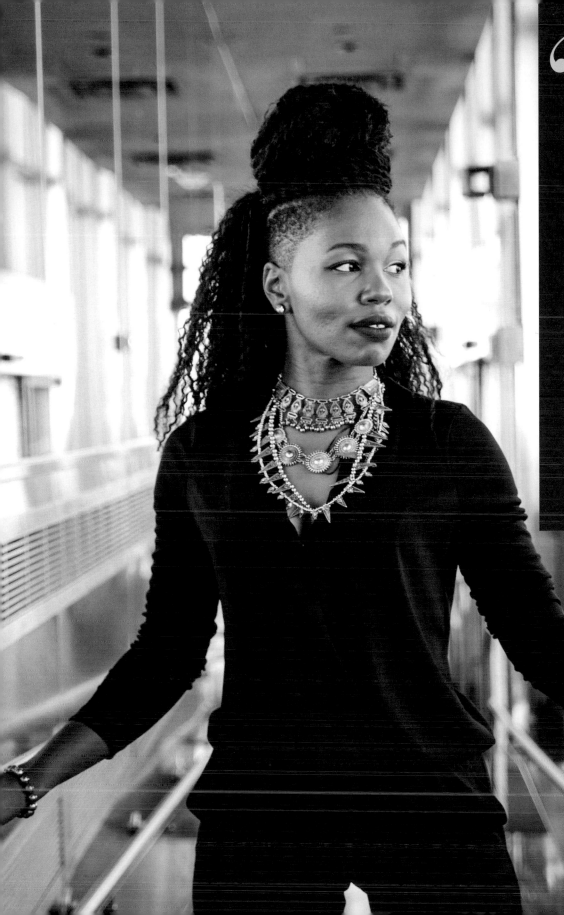

"There are moments where we don't feel cute. We don't feel hot. That's okay. We have different opportunities. It's about being informed."

—Gia Lowe, cofounder and partnerships director for Curly Girl Collective, which connects people and brands

Texture: 4a, normal porosity, coarse, thick

Regimen: When it's warm out, I shampoo once a month and use Kinky-Curly Stellar Strands Conditioner, and SheaMoisture Multi-Vitamin Superfruit Conditioner. I also use Eden Bodyworks Coconut Shea Curl Defining Creme for twist outs and Burgeon Beauty Lab Bloom Oil.

your texture type, the types of styling products you use, how active you are, and even the time of year.

"When you are thinking about shampoos and no-'poos and low-'poos, what you really have to think about is what your hair needs," says influencer Vazquez.

As a general rule of thumb, most curlies don't need to wash their hair every day. One of the main reasons many people wash their hair is because it feels greasy and limp, a result of oils from the scalp spreading over the strands. However, for curlyheads, the curls' natural volume and shape make it difficult for oils to travel down the length of your strands. Depending on your texture type, it may take several days, even weeks, before your hair ever feels oily. For example, wavy hair or fine curly hair usually benefits from cleansing two to three times a week, while thicker curls and coils can usually go a week or more between wash days.

Each curlyhead needs to find the routine that works best for her. Here are some examples from real-life curlies that show a wide variety of cleansing routines:

> **"I cleanse at least once every two weeks with shampoo, and co-wash weekly."**
>
> —CHRISTINA BROWN, 4A, CREATOR OF LOVEBROWNSUGAR.COM.

> **"I don't shampoo anymore. I cleanse with conditioner."**
>
> —AYSHIA COLLIER, 3B, CREATOR OF THE CURLY CROWN

> **"I shampoo once a week, and co-wash every few days."**
>
> —INFLUENCER TIFFANY TATTOOZ, 3C

> **"I mix water, rosemary oil, and a little bit of lavender in a spray bottle— sometimes eucalyptus—and spritz it."**
>
> —KAYLA ANN MCLEOD, WHOSE 4C COILS ARE IN LOCS

Conditioning 101

Conditioner is one of the most important things you can do for your curls. As you've learned, curly textures are naturally dry and can become dehydrated and brittle. It's essential to routinely use products that replace and help retain moisture.

Most curly girls use a variety of conditioners—daily conditioners, detanglers, leave-in conditioners, moisturizers, and deep treatments or masks. While they all moisturize and hydrate, they each are designed to serve a specific purpose. You might use more than one the same day—a daily conditioner in the shower to moisturize and detangle and a leave-in conditioner to seal in moisture. Like all things in the curly world, finding the right products will be trial and error.

"Definitely be patient," says Andrea James, a 3c curly girl who stopped straightening her hair

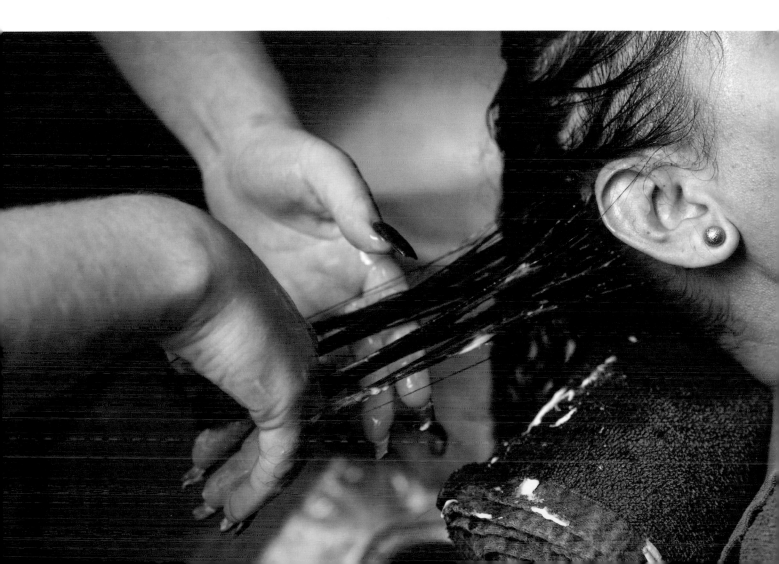

in April 2016. "See what works for you. Just because a product worked for someone else doesn't mean it will work for your hair."

To-Do List: Daily Conditioner & Detangling

Even on days you don't cleanse, you may choose to use a detangler or a daily conditioner. Gentle cleansers, even co-washes, contain moisturizing ingredients, but they are not designed to replace conditioner.

"Conditioners are essential for moisture balance and keeping the hair flexible and stronger. Properly conditioned hair is less vulnerable to dryness and brittle, rough cuticles, and conditioner helps the hair look shinier and full of bounce," says Curly Hair Solutions founder Jonathan Torch.

Daily conditioners usually are designed for daily maintenance and manageability by conditioning the cuticle, making it lie smooth, as well as for enhancing shine and reducing frizz. They typically contain oils, fatty alcohols, and humectants. The purpose of a daily conditioning rinse is to moderately adsorb ingredients onto the surface of your hair.

Detanglers are designed to create slip— the reduction of friction that allows strands of hair to slide past each other (instead of becoming tangled). A detangler enables you to unravel knots and snags with your fingers, wide-tooth comb, or detangling brush. To create this slip, detanglers may contain ingredients like silicones, marshmallow root, slippery elm, or flaxseed.

Whether using a daily conditioner or detangler, be generous with product. Thoroughly cover your entire head. If your curls or waves tend to get weighed down easily, focus on the mid-lengths to the ends and avoid the root area.

You should take full advantage of the slippery effect of your detangler or conditioner; don't be in a rush to rinse your hair without working on any knots or snags first. Your hair is most pliable and easiest to manipulate when it's completely wet and saturated with conditioner. Start from the bottom and work your way up, and use the flow of the shower water to help push out tangles. After your curls are separated and tangle-free, go ahead and rinse.

Many curly girls find a leave-in conditioner to be an indispensable step in their routine. This optional third step in a wash-day routine is helpful if your hair needs a little more moisture after you rinse out your daily conditioner. Generally, leave-in conditioners are lighter and thinner than standard rinse-out conditioners. Some of us prefer creamy leave-ins while others like sprays. Others simply opt for a diluted version of their daily conditioner, by not fully rinsing the daily conditioner out of their hair.

Because some leave-in conditioners offer slight styling properties, they are often used to bridge the gap between conditioning and styling. In fact, some leave-in conditioners—on some hair types—can be used in place of a styling product. You can also use leave-in conditioner as a refresher to get second-day hair or as a mid-afternoon boost.

Oils

Many curlies like to use oils to moisturize their hair. In general oils alone are not moisturizers. The molecules in most oils are too large to be absorbed into the cuticle of the hair, which is why they sit on top of the hair. But there are a few oils that will penetrate the hair shaft and soften the hair from within, including coconut, sunflower, and palm kernel oils.

Erica Douglas, a cosmetic chemist who goes by the name "Sister Scientist," says most oils coat the hair and create a seal, or barrier, to hold moisture in or keep moisture out.

"Using oil on hair that is properly moisturized can help to seal moisture inside the hair, keeping it soft and pliable," Douglas says.

"However, using oil on hair that is already dry creates a barrier on the hair that can reduce or prevent moisture from penetrating after the oil has been applied."

You want to make sure you're using oil after the hair has been properly moisturized with a water-based product. Otherwise, you could be sealing hair that is already dry, and prevent additional moisture from penetrating, actually making it dryer.

Deep-Conditioning: Conditioner on Steroids

Many factors influence your curl's moisture level, including your texture type, the weather and humidity, heat damage, and whether you are in the process of transitioning. Believe it or not, daily conditioning isn't quite enough to keep your curls healthy and soft.

When your curls feel dry, lack shine, lose definition, or become harder to detangle, don't ignore it. Those are signs your hair needs more intense moisture—here's where deep conditioners come into play. Deep conditioners are more heavily concentrated than daily formulas, and they deposit heavier ingredients to hydrate and strengthen your hair.

Looser, finer curls tend to need strengthening treatments, while people with coarser, dryer hair and those who use heat styling and color should use a more intense conditioner, says Torch.

Think proteins, amino acids, and ceramide-rich oils. You can use deep conditioners once a month or more often, depending on your hair type, how dry your hair feels, and the formula. (Some treatments, like ones that contain proteins, can make your hair feel hard or brittle if you overuse them, so always follow the manufacturer's instructions.)

So what's right for your curls? It depends on your texture. Formulas rich in plant oils (coconut, avocado, jojoba, argan, Jamaican Black Castor Oil), butters (shea, mango, cocoa) and moisture-attracting humectants like glycerin, panthenol, and honey can restore moisture and softness. Some hair responds well to hydrolyzed proteins (vegetable, soy, quinoa, rice, and keratin) amino acids (silk), or keratin protein, which can help strengthen and fortify curls.

Want to give your deep treatment more power? Leave it on for at least 30 minutes and add heat or steam using a hot towel, steamy shower, a steamer, a heat cap, or dry hood. These techniques help your cuticle expand and allow the ingredients to penetrate your strands.

Not everyone needs a heavily moisturizing deep conditioner. Torch cautions, "Some curly hair can hold moisture so much that their hair can take up to 10 hours to dry if it is overly conditioned, leaving them with flat, lifeless curls."

PRE-'POO? THE OTHER 'POO

A "pre-'poo" treatment provides an additional boost of moisture. Pre-'pooing is the practice of applying oil or conditioner to the hair before shampooing or cleansing. In addition to offering additional hydration, a pre-'poo can help prep your hair for detangling. You can leave your pre-'poo in 15 minutes before you shower or even overnight, depending on what your hair needs.

Elizabeth Almonte, a 3b curly, pre-'poos with olive oil a half hour before washing. She heats up olive oil and adds a little honey. The olive oil moisturizes while the honey hydrates and attracts moisture, she says. She divides her hair into four sections and applies the oil directly to the hair, adding a little at a time and focusing on her ends while staying away from her roots.

"It makes my ends more manageable and less frizzy and makes my hair stronger, preventing breakage," she says.

STYLING/FINISHING

A stylist once told me, "No styling product, no style."

For many of us curly girls, it's nearly impossible to get definition and frizz control without styling product. The question becomes: What type of styling product or products should you use?

If you get 20 curlies in a room—even if we all have the same texture—we probably each use different styling products. It's all about personal preference. Some of us like a little crunch to hold their curls, while others prefer products with little, if any, hold. Some like the control of a cream; others like gels. Many use a combination of several products—a practice called "cocktailing."

As with many curly topics, there is controversy over styling products, especially when it comes to silicones—also known as "cones." The purpose of silicone is to coat the hair with a micro-fine layer of conditioners that creates sheen, reduces friction, and prevents tangles and breakage. Silicone can also prevent frizz by creating a barrier to humidity.

There are many types of silicones—some water-soluble and some non-water-soluble. Those who follow a no-'poo method avoid non-water-soluble silicones, which can cause buildup over a period of time and may require cleansing with a sulfate-based shampoo to remove.

Ultimately your styling routine will depend on your texture and the style you're going for. A wavy who wants a "beachy wave" look will use completely different products than a coily-haired woman who is doing a twist out.

"Don't feel like you need to nail down a specific routine," says curly hair expert Brianne Prince of the Brianne Prince Salon in Mason, Ohio. "It can vary from day to day. Be creative and go for it, and as needs arise, come up with a creative solution."

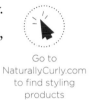

Go to NaturallyCurly.com to find styling products

CURLTALK: PRODUCT COCKTAILS

Many of us spend our lives searching for that one unicorn product—the one that provides everlasting moisture, shine, frizz-less texture that lasts five-days straight and feels soft to the touch. But for those who are still looking, there is a way to get exactly what you want, when you want it—cocktailing.

Cocktailing enables us to customize our regimen by layering styling products. Sometimes one product doesn't give you the benefits of two or three. You may need the hold of a gel but the moisture of a leave-in conditioner.

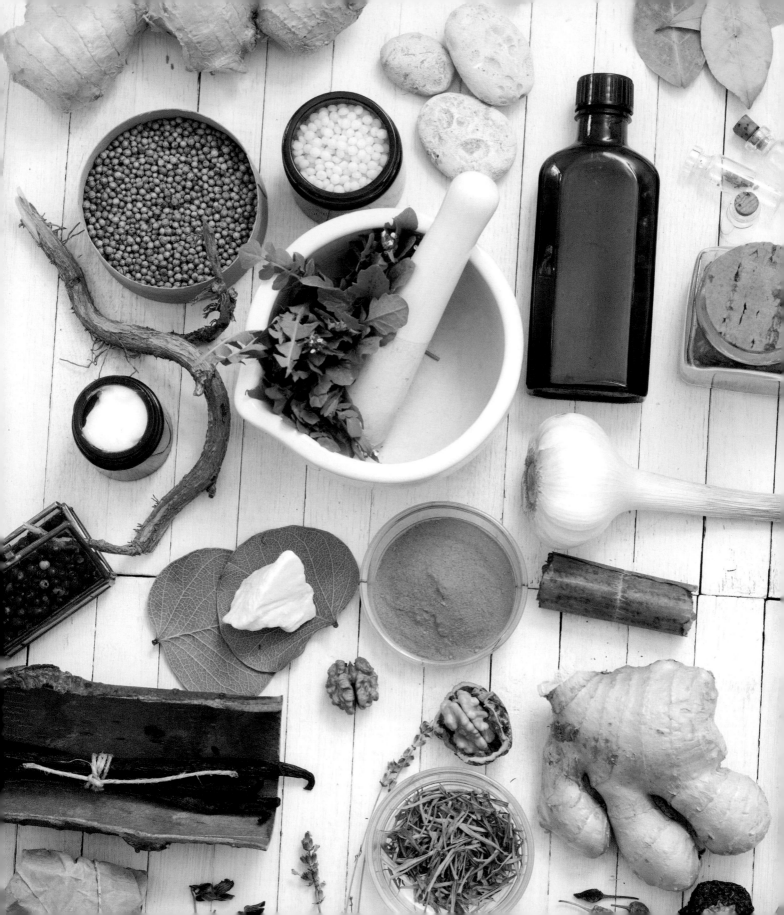

MIXING IT TOGETHER: HOMEMADE TREATMENTS

Some of the best treatments for curly hair can be made from ingredients in your own kitchen.

Here are some favorites from NaturallyCurly mixtresses.

SNOWYMOON'S MOISTURE TREATMENT

Ingredients

4 parts conditioner ('cone-free; I used Giovanni 50/50)

1 part aloe vera gel

1 part honey (warmed 10 seconds)

Oil (optional; I used coconut)

Directions

I used ½ cup of conditioner, 2 tablespoons each of honey and aloe vera gel, and 1 teaspoon of coconut oil—this yielded more than enough for one use. I placed the remainder in a clean, airtight container. You can either warm it all together or warm just the honey and then add the remaining ingredients. I just warmed about 10 seconds.

Be careful not to warm for too long. Mix all ingredients together and place in freshly washed hair with excess water squeezed out. Leave in 30-60 minutes, rinse, and style as usual. Can use with or without heat.

YOGURT HAIR MASK

Ingredients

1 cup of yogurt

2 tablespoons of honey

4 tablespoons of olive oil

2 vitamin E gel capsules

Directions

Mix it up and apply to your hair. Put it up in a shower cap for 30 minutes and wash out.

= natural

PEPPERMINT PRE-'POO

Ingredients

1–2 tablespoons of olive oil or coconut oil 🌿

5–10 drops of peppermint oil 🌿

Directions

Using a spoonful of coconut oil or olive oil, mix in 5 or so drops of peppermint oil. Get your hands wet with the mixture and massage into your scalp. Make sure to rub the mixture through to the end of your strands.

MOISTURIZING DEEP CONDITIONER

Ingredients

2 tablespoons of baking soda

2 tablespoons of olive oil (or your favorite hair oil) 🌿

1 cup of your favorite conditioner

Optional: add a few drops of your favorite scented essential oil

Directions

Mix all ingredients together. Apply to clean hair section by section, working through to the ends. (Be careful of the scalp, since baking soda is abrasive.) Put on shower cap and leave for at least 30 minutes. Rinse thoroughly with warm water and continue with your styling routine.

GREEN TEA VINEGAR RINSE

Ingredients

1 green tea bag

1 cup of water 🌿

1 tablespoon of vinegar (I used non-fruit; ACV is also okay—whatever you have at hand.) 🌿

Directions

Make sure your hair is tangle free. I prefer mine oiled in advance before water washing. Make one cup of green tea. Add the vinegar. Allow the mixture to cool. Pour the mixture on your wet hair. Let it sit in your hair for about ten minutes. Wash off with cold water.

SUPER MAYO DEEP-CONDITIONING TREATMENT

Ingredients

1 cup of real mayo

1 egg

2 tablespoons of extra virgin olive oil

2 tablespoons of extra virgin coconut oil

1 tablespoons of apple cider vinegar

2 tablespoons of honey

1 tablespoon of shea butter

Directions

Combine all ingredients and mix well, either by hand or in a blender. After hair has been washed thoroughly, apply this mixture to hair in sections (or whichever way you prefer). Cover with a plastic cap. If using a heat source (dryer, steamer, etc.), leave on for 20–45 minutes and rinse thoroughly. If using without a heat source, leave hair covered for 1–2 hours prior to rinsing.

LEAVE-IN COCONUT CREAM

Ingredients

2 tablespoons of coconut oil

2 tablespoons of shea butter (raw)

5–10 large drops of honey

You can add oils if you want (tea tree, avocado, jojoba, grape seed, etc., to name a few)

Directions

Melt coconut oil, shea butter, and honey in the microwave for 15–30 seconds or on top of stove for about 2–5 minutes. Pour into a bowl and stir until well blended, then pour into a dark glass container with lid and put in the freezer for about 5–10 minutes. After it hardens you can take out and store in your bathroom! Works wonderfully on my hair. Hopefully it will do the same for you.

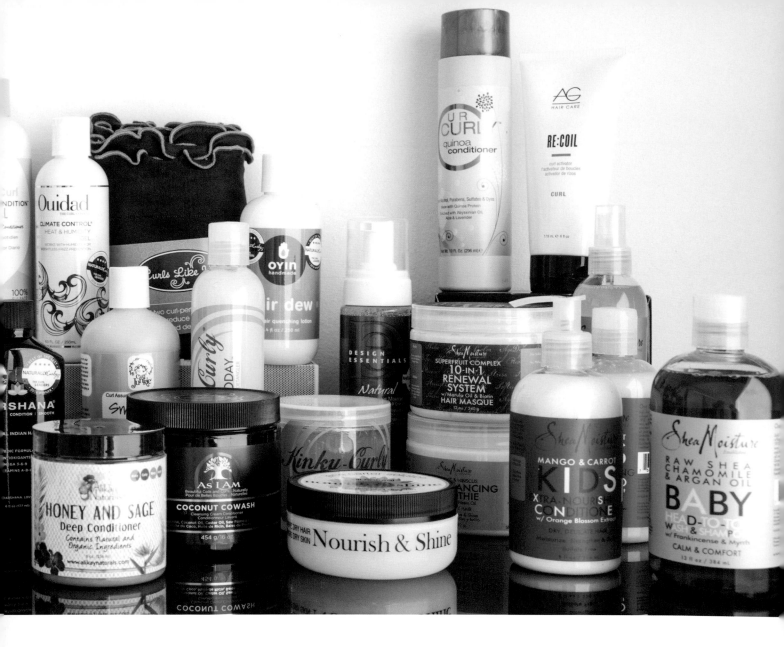

NATURALLYCURLY'S PRODUCT HALL OF FAME

Ever wonder about those Holy Grail products that just keep on knocking our socks off? Looking for products that are loved and recommended by NaturallyCurly community members and editors alike? These curly, coily, and wavy hair products keep making our annual lists—"Editors' Choice" (our editors select their favorites by texture type) and "Best of the Best" (our readers select their favorites), sometimes multiple years in a row!

Go to NaturallyCurly. com to see the latest winners

CLEANSERS

- Jessicurl Hair Cleansing Cream
- Kinky-Curly Come Clean
- SheaMoisture Raw Shea Butter Moisture Retention Shampoo
- As I Am Coconut Cleansing Co-Wash Conditioner
- MopTop Clarifying Rescue Treatment
- DevaCurl No-Poo Quick Cleanser
- Eden Bodyworks Peppermint Tea Tree Shampoo
- NYC Curls The Cleanser

CONDITIONERS

- Kinky-Curly Knot Today
- Karen's Body Beautiful Sweet Ambrosia Leave in Conditioner
- DevaCurl One Condition
- Aubrey Organics Honeysuckle Rose Moisturizing Conditioner
- MopTop Daily Conditioner
- Paul Mitchell Curls Full-Circle Leave-In Treatment
- Joico K-Pak Reconstructor Conditioner
- Oyin Handmade Hair Dew
- U R Curly Quinoa Conditioner
- Nubian Heritage Honey & Black Seed Heat-Protect Leave-In Conditioning Cream

- Amika Perk Up Dry Shampoo
- SheaMoisture Superfruit Complex 10-in-1 Renewal System Masque
- Alikay Naturals Honey & Sage Deep Conditioner
- Obia Natural Hair Care Curl Hydration Spray
- Obia Naturals Curl Moisture Cream
- SheaMoisture Raw Shea Butter Extra-Moisture Transitioning Milk

CURL REFRESHER

- Jessicurl Awe Inspiraling Spray

STYLING PRODUCTS

- Kinky-Curly Curling Custard
- Herbal Essences Totally Twisted Curl Boosting Mousse
- Miss Jessie's Curly Pudding
- AG Re:coil
- SheaMoisture Organic Coconut & Hibiscus Curl Enhancing Smoothie
- Jane Carter Wrap & Roll
- AG Beach Bomb
- Ampro Olive Oil Gel
- Jane Carter Nourish & Shine
- Design Essentials Natural Curl Enhancing Mousse
- Pantene Pro-V Curl Defining Mousse

- Curl Junkie Curl Assurance Smoothing Lotion
- Paul Mitchell Fast Form
- Eden Bodyworks Coconut Curl Defining Crème
- Amika Undone Texture Spray
- Ecoco Ecostyling Olive Oil Gel
- Curly Hair Solutions Curl Keeper Original

OIL

- Ouidad Mongongo Oil
- Darshana Natural Indian Hair Oil
- AG The Oil

FINISHER

- SheaMoisture Raw Shea Butter Reconstructive Finishing Elixir
- Oyin Handmade Burnt Sugar Pomade

TOOLS

- CHI Original Flat Iron
- Hair Therapy Wrap
- Scent-Sation Spa Satin Pillowcase
- CurlFormers
- Denman D3 Brush
- Curls Like Us Curl Cloths
- Amika Tourmaline Clip-Free Curler

VITAMINS

- Nature's Bounty Optimal Solutions Extra Strength Hair, Skin and Nails Argan Oil Infused Multivitamin
- Hairfinity Healthy Hair Vitamins

FOR KIDS

- SheaMoisture Kids Line

BRAND

- SheaMoisture

COLLECTION

- L'Oreal Paris Evercurl (Cleansing Balm, Hydracharge Leave-in Cream, Hydracharge Conditioner, Sculpt & Hold Cream-Gel)

To check out all of our most popular Hall of Fame winners, please go to NaturallyCurly. com/hall-of-fame

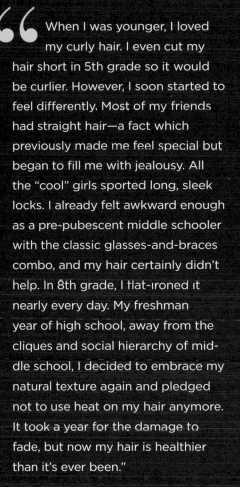

> "When I was younger, I loved my curly hair. I even cut my hair short in 5th grade so it would be curlier. However, I soon started to feel differently. Most of my friends had straight hair—a fact which previously made me feel special but began to fill me with jealousy. All the "cool" girls sported long, sleek locks. I already felt awkward enough as a pre-pubescent middle schooler with the classic glasses-and-braces combo, and my hair certainly didn't help. In 8th grade, I flat-ironed it nearly every day. My freshman year of high school, away from the cliques and social hierarchy of middle school, I decided to embrace my natural texture again and pledged not to use heat on my hair anymore. It took a year for the damage to fade, but now my hair is healthier than it's ever been."

—Emma Seaborn, high school student

Texture: 3a/3b, high porosity, fine, thin

Regimen: I typically use a clarifying shampoo, such as Quidad Superfruit Renewal Clarifying Cream Shampoo, followed by a deep conditioner (my current favorite is OBIA Naturals' Babassu Deep Conditioner; it's vegan, natural, and makes my hair super soft!). Lastly, I apply Curlisto Repair Styling Cream, a leave-in conditioner. I wash my hair twice a week, and in-between I use RICH De-frizz and Shine Mist and apply argon oil to my ends.

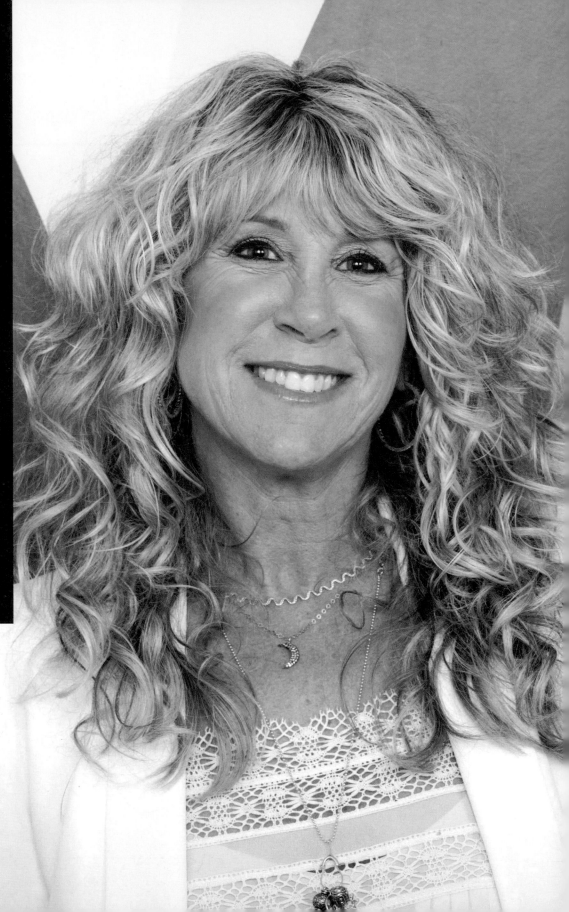

> "Wavy girls don't always realize what their hair is capable of. They often believe their hair is straight, frizzy, unkempt, and frazzled. They typically rely on blow dryers, hot tools, and brushes to prevent it from doing what it's truly capable of. We're guiding the wavy client, just as we're guiding the curly and the super-curly clients."

—Shari Harbinger, cofounder DevaCurl Academy

Texture: 2b, low porosity, fine, medium density

Regimen: I cleanse with Deva-Curl Delite Low-Poo, DevaCurl Delite, or DevaCurl Original One Condition, and style with DevaCurl Frizz Free Volumizing Foam and DevaCurl Light Defining Gel.

Chapter 5

FROM CURL KABOBS TO PLOPPING—

TRIED-AND-TRUE CURL-STYLING TECHNIQUES

Each curly's styling routine is as unique as her fingerprint, honed over years of trial and error, and most likely modified on a regular basis.

To style her 3b curls, Morgan Marshall starts in the shower, running her fingers through her hair to detangle. After the shower, she gently pats her hair with a towel and applies oil throughout her hair. She then parts her hair and applies gel on each side. After that, she scrunches with a microfiber glove, applying her styling mousse and scrunching again—all while her head is flipped upside down. Then she uses a diffuser to completely dry her curls. Once dry, she puts more oil in and finishes with a hairspray. Marshall has used her "Tame the Mane" routine for three years.

Nasstassia Davy's go-to style for her 4b coils is a twist out. She washes her hair, and then separates it into four sections. Then she applies a combination of leave-in conditioner, styling cream, and oil to smaller sections. She does 5 to 6 medium-sized 2-strand twists per section. Davy keeps her hair in the twists until they're completely dry—usually a day or two. Then she applies oil to her hands and unravels the twists from end to root, gently separating them. For the finishing touches, she uses an Afro pick to full up her roots and applies an edge-control gel around her hairline.

Maranda Moody is a big fan of plopping for her 3a loose curls, a technique she discovered on NaturallyCurly. She scrunches in gel and then ties her head up in a T-shirt and sleeps in it overnight. In the morning, she diffuses it for exactly three minutes.

"You could have the best haircut in the world, but if you don't know how to style it, it's going to go all over the place," says Ouidad. "You need to understand how to reset the curl pattern back to its shape."

In so many ways, you have a big advantage over your friends and family with straight hair when it comes to styling. By using different techniques, you can easily get completely different looks. Whether it is elongating curls, defining waves, or creating big, beautiful Afros, there is a technique for you—many created by NaturallyCurly's community.

For example, curly hair stylist Brianne Prince developed her "Plopping with a Veil Net" technique at her Mason, Ohio, salon when she noticed it was taking a long time for her wavier clients' hair to dry, even under a dryer hood. She saw a veil net in a store—the kind of nets used by older women for their roller sets—and saw it as the ideal replacement for the towel or T-shirt usually used to plop.

"The idea is to let the air flow through the net to let the hair dry quicker," Prince says. "You can take the diffuser off the dryer and still not disturb the hair. With curly hair, some of the best ideas come from play."

SO MANY STYLING TECHNIQUES, SO LITTLE TIME

There are so many different ways to create looks for your hair. Here are a few, and you can find how-to videos for all of these styles on NaturallyCurly.com

---

KEY STYLING TOOLS:

- Wide-tooth comb for detangling
- Microfiber towel/glove or T-shirt to remove moisture without causing frizz
- A pick
- Flexible rods/curlers
- A diffuser or hood dryer to gently dry and set curls
- Duckbill clips for volume at the roots
- Water bottle or mister

The Smaster

Created by CurlTalk user Smasters467, the basic idea behind the method is that adding in a curl enhancer product to your hair when it's half dried will help encourage curls more than when applied soaking wet.

1. Apply your products as you normally would and diffuse your hair.

2. Once your hair is about 50 percent dry, turn off your diffuser and move to a sink.

3. Wet your hands and use about a quarter-sized amount of curl enhancer gel on your hair.

4. Gently scrunch the gel into your hair. You should be cautious not to break up any clumps that may have started to form.

5. Dry your hair again to your preference. There are some differing opinions about whether to use hot heat or low or warm heat. It depends on what works for your hair; drying on hot heat will help encourage your hair to shrink and create more defined curls, which is ideal for wavies. Using a warm or cool setting will give more elongation, which may be ideal for coilier textures.

Scrunching

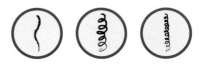

This classic method enhances your curl pattern.

1. Add leave-in conditioner to freshly washed and conditioned waves, then gently squeeze out excess water.

2. Apply mousse, gel, or sea salt spray to your hair in sections.

3. Next, scrunch by cupping a section in your palm and squeezing until there is no more water dripping. Repeat for all sections.

4. Once your waves are dry and set, you can coat your palms with a little oil or serum and scrunch them once more to break the cast, or "scrunch the crunch."

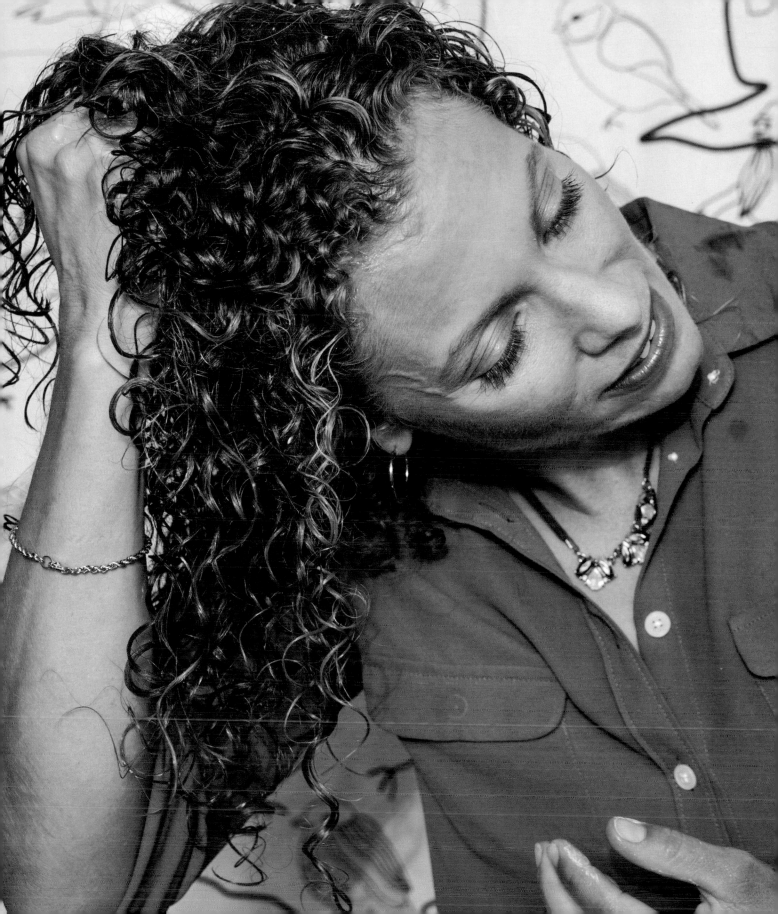

Diffusing

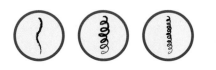

Diffusers attach to your blow-dryer and gently disperse airflow over a larger area so it doesn't disturb your hair pattern or create frizz. Diffusing can create more curl definition, add volume, and refresh your style.

1. After washing and conditioning, use a microfiber towel or a T-shirt to remove water from hair and then apply gel or mousse.

2. To dry, tilt your hair sideways or upside down and place sections of your hair into the bowl of the diffuser.

3. Continue until your hair is 80 to 90 percent dry. Gently scrunch, then mist a layer of sea salt or texturizing spray as a finishing touch.

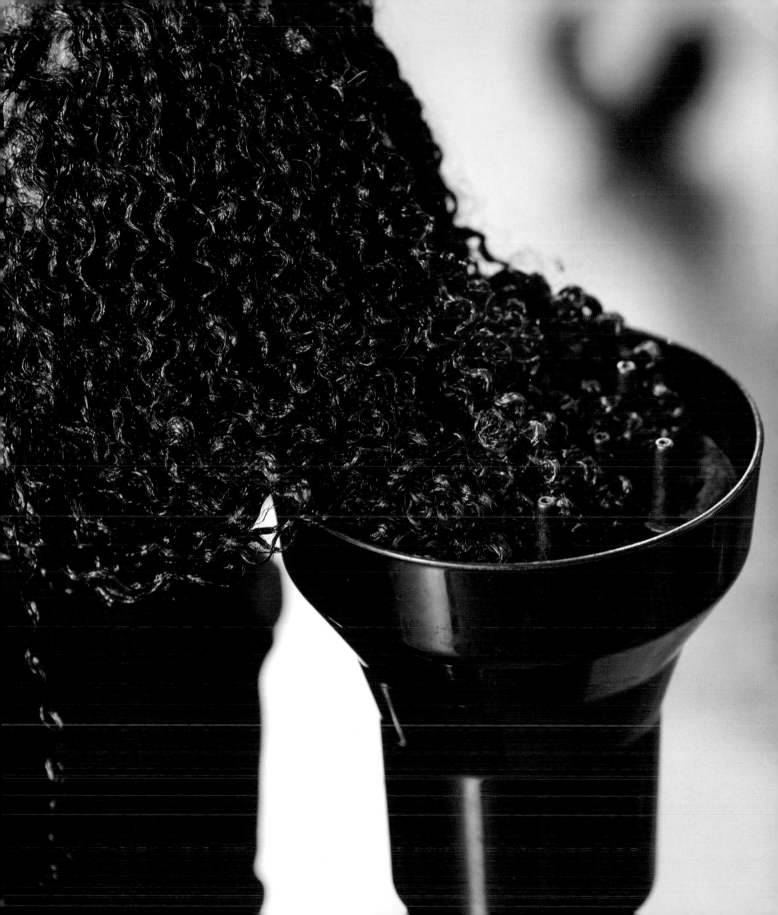

Run & Swift

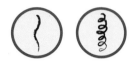

This technique was developed by curl expert Christo of New York's Christo Fifth Avenue to encourage curl formation.

1. Apply styling product to hands and run your fingers through each section of the hair as if it were a comb, in order to distribute your product equally.

2. Shake each section quickly in a left to right motion.

3. Either diffuse or air-dry.

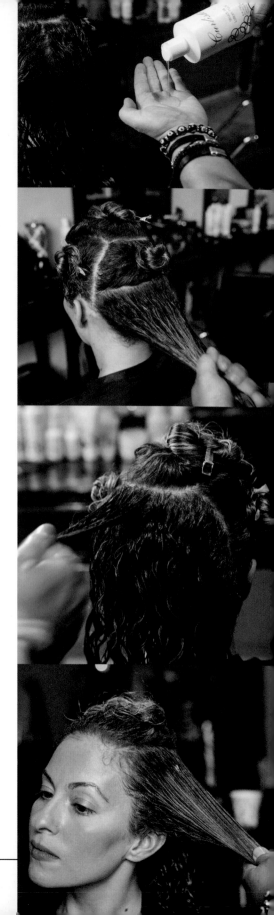

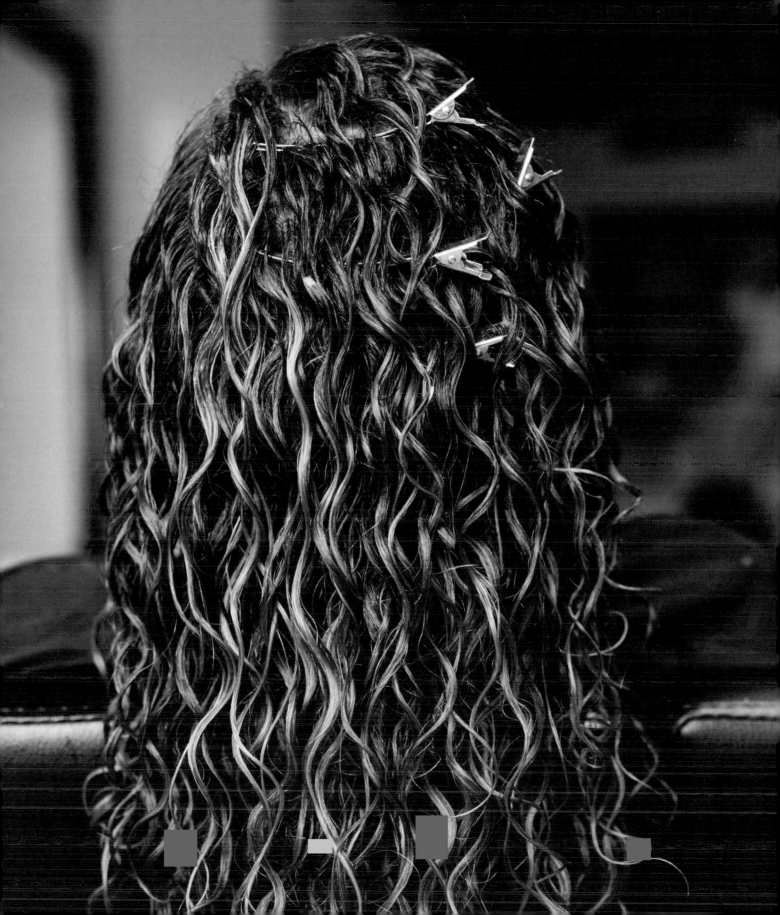

The Rake & Shake

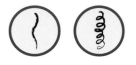

This technique was created by Ouidad to define curls and ensure even product application.

1. With gel in your palm, rub your hands together and grab your hair in sections from the root.

2. Spread your fingers apart and then slide your fingers through the length of your hair to the ends to recreate the curl pattern. At the ends, lightly grasp the hair between your fingers and give the strands a little shake.

3. Then, take duck clips, put them on their side, and gently slide them across your scalp to clip the hair and lift the root up, allowing the curls to cascade down.

Clumping

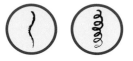

You get shapely, well-defined curls when your hair forms and dries in chunky groups or clusters. The key is to encourage the strands to cluster together during styling.

1. Start with freshly washed and conditioned hair. Then add a moisturizing cream, serum, or leave-in conditioner, followed by a defining product like a gel or mousse.

2. Scrunch your hair as you apply your styling products to help your curls stick together.

3. Blot away extra product with a microfiber towel or T-shirt.

4. Air-dry or diffuse without disturbing the curl pattern.

Super-Soaker Method for Clumping

CurlTalker Rudeechick came up with this new method for clumping. She found that when she scrunched in product, it resulted in massive volume and separated curls.

1. Wash and condition hair and rake through a leave-in.

2. Brush a base coat of styling product through hair, first at the nape and then at the back of the head. (Use products with slip and use good-quality brushes and combs.)

3. Use the brush to part hair and do a final brushing of the crown.

4. Lean over the sink to one side, cupping hands under the running water and gently scrunching palmfuls of water into the hair. Repeat to the other side. (Don't scrunch firm and tight, but slowly and softly to thoroughly soak the hair.)

5. At this point, the hair is more soaked than it would normally be when you step out of the shower. Scrunch in the gel of choice and plop (5–10 minutes).

6. Air-dry or diffuse.

Pin Curls

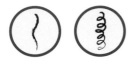

By setting your hair into small twists or braids, you can encourage lasting curl formation.

1. Apply mousse or gel to damp hair; then divide your hair into six to eight sections.

2. Twist each section and pin into place with a bobby pin.

3. Diffuse or allow your hair to air-dry before unraveling.

4. Give your hair a shake and fluff out the roots for volume.

Finger Curls/Twirling

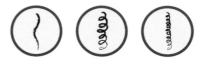

You can use this method for sections with less definition or apply it to your whole head.

1. Apply your preferred styling products to cleansed and conditioned hair.

2. Wind small sections around your finger to create curly coils.

3. Gently let it go and repeat on remaining sections. Allow your curls to dry without further touching your hair.

Skip Curls

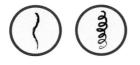

Enhance your natural spiral pattern with this method created by curl expert Jonathan Torch.

1. Finger comb a strong-hold gel through your hair and remove any tangles.

2. Take a small section and twist it around your finger from the root to end.

3. Slide your finger out of the twist and grasp the end, then swing or "skip" the strand like a jump rope. Gently release the curl.

4. Repeat method for the rest of your hair. Finally, flip your hair upside down and back to add some volume, then allow to air-dry.

Curl Kabobs

When clipping became difficult for curl expert Brianne Prince of Brianne Prince Salon, she invented a new gravity-defying technique: curl kebabs. For this technique, Brianne recommends using anything that's long, thin, and not blunt at the ends so as not to disturb the curl pattern. Kebab skewers, pencils, chopsticks, rattail combs, or anything you have in this shape will work.

1. Take two skewers and slide them towards each other at the crown of the head, slightly lifting the roots and crossing the skewers.

2. Continue to do this, moving backwards away from the face. Brianne uses four pairs of skewers, but do what works for you.

Plopping

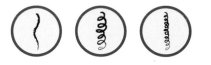

You need to use a long-sleeved T-shirt for this type of wet set to absorb excess water.

1. Wash and condition hair as usual.

2. Apply your leave-in conditioner or moisturizer while hair is still damp.

3. Spread a large cotton T-shirt on a flat surface, with the sleeves closest to you.

4. Hang your head forward so that your hair falls in front of your face and lands in the center of the shirt.

5. Slowly lower your head so that all your hair falls in layers onto the shirt. Think of pouring cake batter.

6. Grab the bottom corners of the T-shirt and bring the bottom edge of the T-shirt across your forehead. Grip the corners in the back of your head to hold the T-shirt in place.

7. Grab the top of the shirt, bring it over the back of your head and tuck the neckline down to the base of your neck. This should cause the sleeves to move to the side of your head.

8. Bring the sleeves around to the front of your forehead and tie. Tuck in any loose bits of t-shirt so that everything is secure.

9. The next morning, undo the t-shirt.

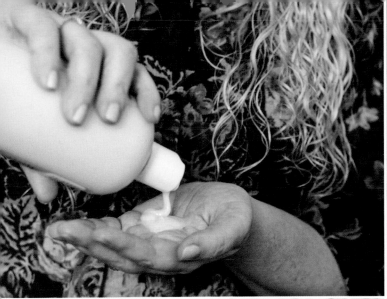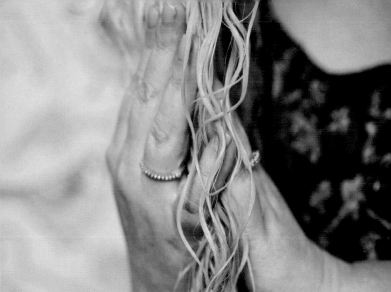
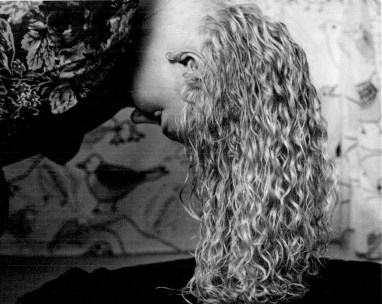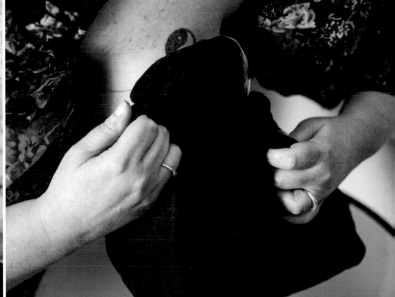
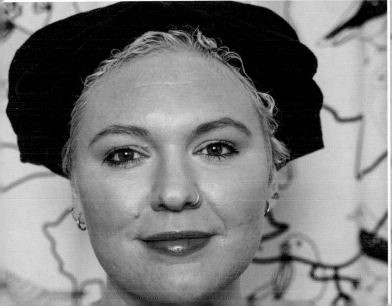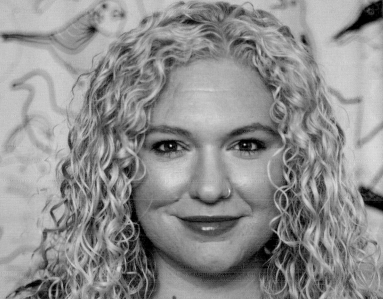

Shingling

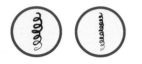

Shingling is a styling method developed by Miss Jessie's salon to manually elongate curls and create definition. It is called "shingling" because it looks like flat shingles layered on each other.

1. Wash, condition, and detangle your hair.

2. Separate your hair into twists.

3. Spray your hair to get it damp.

4. Undo a twist.

5. Rake a styling product through the twist you just untwisted.

6. Repeat through the rest of the twists.

Banding

This involves the use of hair ties or ponytail holders to gently stretch the hair by holding the curls in an elongated position as they dry.

1. Wash, condition, and detangle hair.

2. Apply your favorite leave-in conditioner and styler, and section your hair into medium-sized, workable sections, depending on length and density.

3. Wrap a hair tie or ponytail holder twice around the base of each section (at the scalp) and then use additional ties to wrap every 2"–3" along the length of each section, down to the ends. Repeat until all sections are banded.

4. Allow the hair to dry thoroughly before removing the ponytail holders. Depending on your texture, you may end up with looser curls or waves or even a blowout-like straightness.

Wash 'n Go

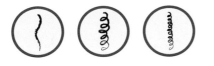

This low-maintenance technique is pretty simple. This is a universal styling technique.

1. Wash your hair and condition your hair.

2. Apply styling products to dripping-wet hair.

3. Allow hair to dry naturally without manipulation.

Bantu Knot Out

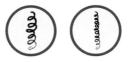

This protective styling method originates from African tribes and involves twisting hair into small knots to create defined curls.

1. Divide freshly washed, detangled, and moisturized hair into small, triangular sections.

2. Twist each section to create a little bun and secure with ouchless bands or bobby pins. You can wear the knots as a style and then, for another look, once hair is fully dry remove the knots and gently separate with hair oil.

Pineapple

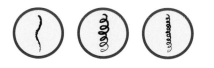

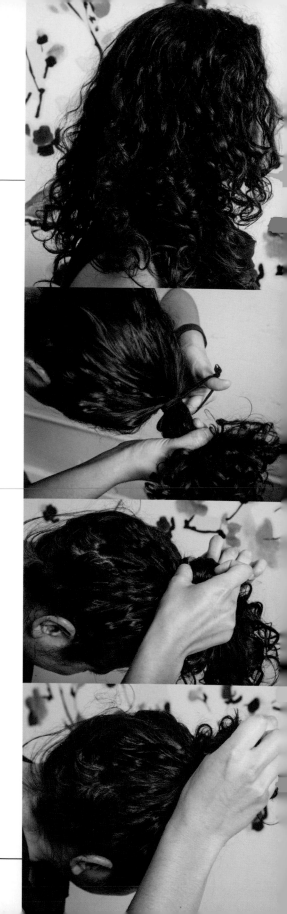

Protect your curls from getting smashed and bent while you sleep.

1. Gently pile the hair on the center of your head and secure with a loose scrunchie before bed. If you have shorter hair, use two or three scrunchies to make a few high ponytails.

2. For extra protection, you can also wrap hair in a satin scarf or sleep on a satin pillowcase.

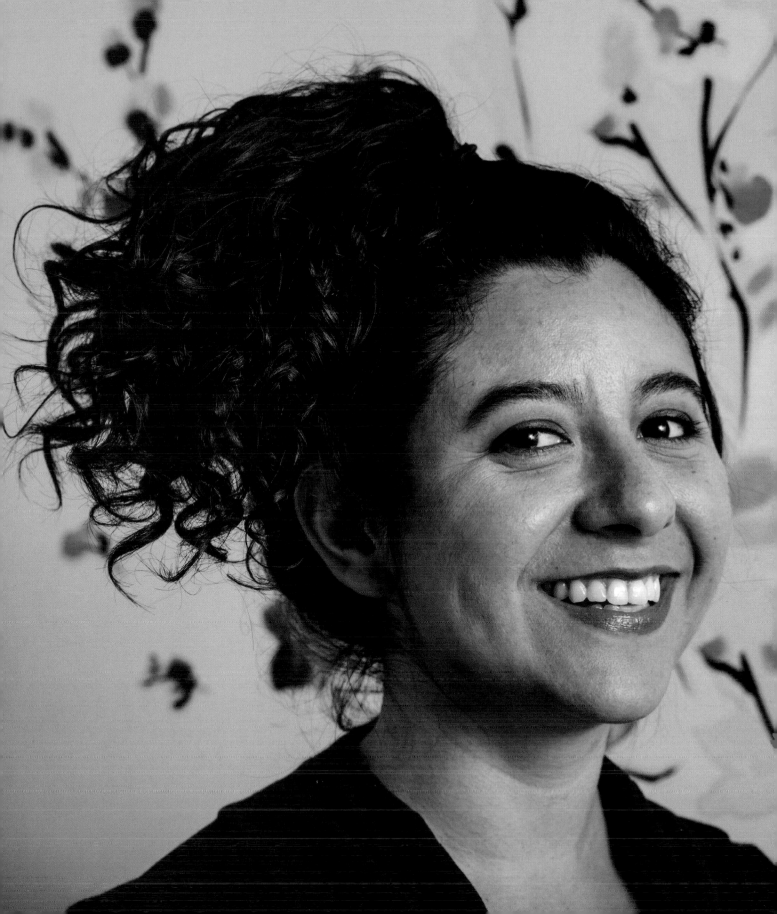

Twist Out or Braid Out

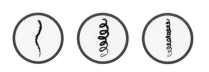

These techniques are used for curlies who have less-distinct curls, even when the hair is in a wet state. A twist out is when you intertwine two clusters of hair like a rope to help stretch out and elongate your curl. Braid outs are created in the same fashion as two-strand twists, but the sectioned hair is braided instead of twisted.

1. Part your hair in sections and apply your favorite moisturizer and styler.

2. Create small two-strand twists or braids.

3. For more polished ends, use flexi rollers or curl the ends around your finger to ensure the ends are smooth.

4. Leave the twists or braids in overnight or diffuse.

5. Gently unravel and wear loose or style into an updo.

Afro

You can create an Afro style by teasing out a second-day twist out or wash 'n go.

1. Use a cream or gloss to lightly separate the curls and fluff up the roots with your fingers.

2. Working in sections, use a pick to create desired level of volume.

3. Finish with oil spray if you want sheen.

Finger Coils

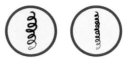

Similar to finger curls/twisting. This method helps create uniform curls so it's good for uneven curl patterns, frizz, or patches that refuse to curl.

1. Separate freshly washed and conditioned hair into small sections.

2. Apply a moisturizer or leave-in, then add a layer of gel or styling cream.

3. Stretch and twirl each section until the hair forms a coil down to the scalp.

4. Repeat for entire head.

5. You can leave the coils "as is" for a couple days, if desired, and then gently separate them for a new look.

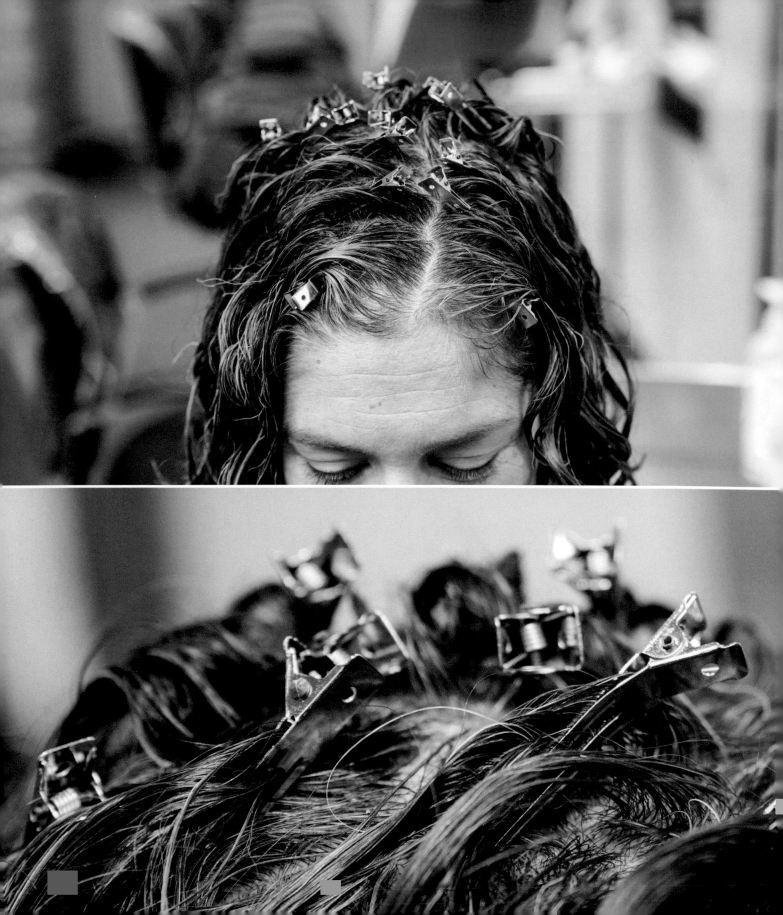

Clipping

Clipping your hair is a great way to give it instant lift at the roots where it might otherwise be flat. Curly hair looks great, but has a tendency to fall flat at the top. Clipping enables you to offset gravity's force and add body back to limp roots quickly.

1. Apply your favorite styling product to wet hair, or for dry or second-day hair, use a mixture of water and conditioner in a spray bottle.

2. With wet hair, section off around five or six sections of the hair on each side of the hairline.

3. Take a clip—many use duckbill clips or jaw clips—and clip it right at the roots of each section, along the part.

4. Diffuse the hair for a few minutes, paying special attention to the roots and crown area.

5. Remove the clips, flip your head upside down and shake your hair without touching it.

Bun Drying

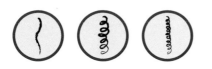

This technique involves using a topknot to elongate the texture.

1. Start by cleansing, conditioning, and using a wide-tooth comb to detangle (The wide-tooth comb helps clump the curls together.)

2. Blot your hair dry with a basic cotton T-shirt instead of a towel. Blotting will remove any excess water and the T-shirt will prevent frizz.

3. Gently apply a styler all over the hair.

4. Pull hair onto the top of the head and secure in a loose topknot. Leave the hair in a topknot until halfway dry (the roots and back will still feel wet).

5. Take your hair down from the topknot and allow it to air-dry the rest of the way while the hair is down and loose.

6. You can use your fingers to lightly loosen the roots if they look flat or too clumped together as they dry.

Roller Sets

These can be done with rubber rods, flexible rollers, styling sticks, or CurlFormer. They provide a heat-free way to create defined curls. Roller sets allow you to change the texture of any curl pattern or density, depending upon the size of the rod, stick, or CurlFormer.

1. Start with washed and detangled hair.

2. Section your hair into four sections, and then, starting at the nape, section into subsections no more than two inches in diameter.

3. Cover each section with a moisturizer and styling gel.

4. Now, you can use one of three techniques. No. 1: Hold the roller near the root and begin winding the hair around the remainder of the roller. No. 2: Hold the roller on your ends, wind it up toward the root, and fold to secure. No. 3: Apply CurlFormers per manufacturer's directions.

5. Dry hair—you can sleep in them or use a dryer—before removing rods, one at a time.

6. Pick or shake out the curls.

10 TIPS FOR STYLING

1. Cleanse Before Styling

Before styling your hair, it is important to wash out all the leftover products that might be in your hair. Prior to styling, start with a clean, freshly washed head of hair—a clean canvas to apply new product and create your fresh style.

2. Use a Leave-In Conditioner

The key to a frizz-free style is moisture. Moisturizing the hair will not only help its overall health, but it will also keep your frizz at bay.

3. Check the Forecast First

Go to NaturallyCurly. com to use Frizz Forecast

It's important to customize your regimen during different seasons. If it's humid and hot outside, stay away from products with glycerin in them, and instead stick to anti-humectants. Check out NaturallyCurly's Frizz Forecast to find out what the weather has in store for your hair and what types of products to use for your texture type and style.

4. Section Your Curls

Several curlies complain that their hair turns out differently across different areas of the head. The problem often lies in uneven product application. Section your hair with clips to ensure even product application. Apply product in sections—the smaller the sections, the better.

5. Soaking Wet Hair Is Best

Many stylists recommend applying hair product when the hair is very wet. Hair product usually reacts better to wet hair because it helps with clumping, which is essential to curl formation.

6. Scrunch Out the Crunch

Is your hair crunchy after styling? A gel cast actually helps to hold the curls in their natural formation until the hair dries while simultaneously protecting the hair from outside elements like wind and humidity. When curls are dry, simply break the cast by lightly scrunching upward. This helps to break up the gel while lifting from the scalp to give the hair height.

7. Air-Dry

Air-dry your curls as often as you can. Your hair will thank you, and you will notice a difference over time in the way your hair dries.

8. Don't Touch

Remember, friction is not your friend. Be careful not to over-manipulate your hair, or you may break up the curls and create frizz. It is best not to touch your hair until it's completely dry.

9. Hold It in Place

If your hair is especially prone to frizz, hairspray can be your friend. And a growing number of hair care product manufacturers have created fast-drying formulas that block humidity, add shine, and keep your curls intact.

10. Refresh Those Curls

If your curls and waves are looking a little droopy, you can spritz in one of the many curl revitalizers on the market. Or spray them with a mix of leave-in conditioner and water. This will reactivate the styling product and redefine your curls.

TOP TIPS FOR SECOND-DAY HAIR

Second-day hair is the ability to retain a hairstyle from one day to the next without completely restyling it. We have watched, read, and listened to countless curlies share their second-day hair tips. While every head of curls is unique, we did manage to find some major similarities between almost all of them. Here are some ways to achieve beautiful second-day hair.

It Starts with First-Day Hair

If you are wanting second-, third-, or even fourth-day hair, it all starts with Day 1. You must properly cleanse, condition, and deep condition your hair. You can't do that after the fact.

Protect It

Bedtime can be the enemy for second-day hair. That's because the friction created by the pillow can create frizz and flattened hair. You can keep your hair in place by putting it up in a pineapple or using a satin bonnet or Loc Soc (a hair accessory that can be used to keep your locs in place at night). You may have another technique that works well for you. Some curlies simply sleep on a satin pillowcase.

Freshen It Up

Second-day hair does not mean the hair hasn't been primped or altered. It means you aren't starting from scratch. Most curly girls refresh their curls in the morning. You can use a curl fresher or leave-in conditioner. A steamer can also refresh curls.

Accessories Are Your Friend

If you wake up with a frizz halo, put on a colorful headband. Or buy some pretty scarves to wrap around your hair.

Change It Up

Second-day hair does not have to look exactly like first-day hair. You may create an updo, a braid, or a messy bun. The beauty of curls and coils is that they don't have to look precise. They are perfectly imperfect. "The messier the better," says curly hair stylist Brianne Prince. "You don't want a perfect, tight braid with curly hair. Curly hair is eclectic, and it transcends any trends."

STRAIGHT TALK ABOUT STRAIGHTENING

Myleik Teele has been natural for more than 15 years. But being natural doesn't mean she wears her hair curly all the time. On this particular day, for example, she's sporting a short, sleek 'do. The founder of curlBOX—a monthly subscription service for women with curls and coils—calls herself a "straight natural."

"Natural hair is not one thing," she says. "What I like most about wearing my hair like this—once you go natural, your hair doesn't stay in one state. The whole point is to have healthy hair that's free of chemicals. You can be straight, natural, curly, or in-between. The goal is to know you always have options."

Many textured-hair women like the option of wearing their hair straight as well as curly. When they do opt for a sleeker look, we help them do it in a way that doesn't damage the hair.

Irreversible damage can occur when the protein bonds in the hair are permanently altered to the point that the hair does not return to its natural curl pattern, and hair struggles to retain moisture as it once did. If you heat keratin (of which hair is composed) to around 215–235 degrees Celsius (or

I think embracing your texture doesn't mean wearing your hair one way all the time. You can embrace it by wearing it naturally curly sometimes and blowing it out straight other times. Hair is an expression of art. It's an expression of your mood."

—Nancy Twine, founder of Briogeo product line

Texture: 3b formerly 4c, medium porosity, fine, medium density

Regimen: I rotate Briogeo Be Gentle Be Kind Avocado Quinoa Co-wash with Briogeo Curl Charisma Shampoo and Conditioner. If I'm styling curly, I use Curl Charisma Leave-in Cream with the ends sealed with Briogeo Rosarca Oil. Then I layer on Briogeo Curl Charisma Frizz Control Gel and diffuse dry for added definition. If I'm styling straight, I use Briogeo Rosarca Shampoo and Conditioner with Rosacroco Milk Leave-in Spray and Rosacroco Oil on the ends. Then, I blow it out and run it through with a flat iron on medium heat.

> "Natural hair is not one thing. The whole point is to have healthy hair. You can be straight natural, curly, or in between."

—Myleik Teele, founder of curlBOX curl subscription box

Texture: 4b with 3a around the edges, high porosity, fine, medium density

Regimen: SheaMoisture Jamaican Black Castor Oil Deep Conditioner, and a dollop of LouAna All Natural Pure Coconut Oil.

419–455 degrees Fahrenheit), the alpha helix (part of a protein molecule) starts to melt.

Chemicals, such as ammonium thioglycolate, sodium hydroxide, and aldehydes, can also alter the hair's protein bonds, resulting in straighter hair. These are physical changes and are irreversible. Your hair will retain the shape of the changed keratin at a molecular level.

Here are specific steps to take to ensure that you don't permanently damage your hair.

Deep Condition Before and After

If your hair is not protein sensitive, now is a good time to use a mask with added proteins. Protein strengthens and repairs the keratin, therefore giving hair structure and helping it grow longer and stronger. For protein-sensitive curlies—whose hair tends to become dry and hard after using a protein treatment—opt for a conditioner with moisturizing butters and oils. By using a deep conditioner before heat styling, you are helping to strengthen the hair for the process, and using it afterward will rejuvenate your curls.

Reduce Straightening Frequency

There is no rule of thumb, but most curl stylists agree that moderation is best when it comes to straightening. You never know how your curly, coily, or wavy hair will react to the intense heat of flat ironing and drying. Does that mean you should never straighten your hair? Absolutely not. If you're going to straighten, be strategic about it. Rely on wash-and-go and protective styles most of the time, recommends Anthony Dickey, author of *Hair Rules* and founder of a salon and a product line of the same name.

Lower the Temperature

The lower the temperature, the less likely the hair is to experience damage. Usually the rule of thumb is that the thicker the strands, the higher the temperature it takes to straighten them. Most curlies try to stay under 375 or 350 degrees F. The finer the hair, the less heat required to straighten it.

Use a Heat Protectant

Most hair care experts will recommend using some sort of heat protectant, like a heat protection spray, serum, or cream. Heat protectants contain a cationic conditioner such as Quaternium 70 or a polymer such as P/DMAPA Acrylates Copolymer. These ingredients have been proven to prevent damage from high-heat styling tools such as blow-dryers and curling or straightening irons. You want to apply the heat protectant while the hair is damp and before the blow-dry process in order to seal in moisture.

Stretch Before Straightening

If you do opt for a blow-dryer, try the tension method. Extreme heat paired with extreme tension is one of the most effective ways to straighten hair, says curl expert Jonathan Torch. Torch recommends using a round brushing with tension while blasting heat to dry the stretched hair. To set the hair in its straight position, he suggests allowing the hair to cool down, or using the cool setting on your dryer, while keeping the tension. Going over the hair with a flat iron will smooth the hair and get it even straighter, he says.

Blow-Dry on Damp, Not Wet, Hair

If you opt to use the tension method or blow-dryer with comb attachment to stretch your hair prior to straightening, make sure the hair is damp and not wet. Blow-drying wet hair is equivalent to frying the hair—very harsh.

Seek Heat-Free Straightening Alternatives

If you want to learn how to straighten your hair without heat, YouTube is full of roller set and roller wrap tutorials. You may not have the same finish as you would with a flat iron, but you won't have heat damage, either.

TEXTURIZING: FROM SILKENERS TO TEX-LAXING TO KERATIN TREATMENTS

For those curlies who like to go back and forth between their curls and straight hair, there are chemical options that loosen the curl. Unlike traditional relaxers, they don't permanently straighten the hair.

Keratin treatments have been the most popular option. They use a combination of keratin and chemicals (the use of formaldehyde in some treatments has been highly controversial) to break up the strong bonds within the hair shaft. The hair is then flat ironed to seal the cuticle. The combination of formaldehyde, heat, and compression all react with the keratin in the hair, loosening the curl. A keratin treatment will not leave you with pin-straight hair but rather relaxes the tightness of your waves.

Another popular option is texlaxing. Texlaxing is the term used for deliberately under-processing hair during a relaxer procedure. The relaxer is not allowed to fully straighten the hair, allowing it to retain more of its elasticity and thickness than fully straightened relaxed hair.

Texlaxing is achieved by using either a lye or no-lye relaxer that is weakened by adding a small amount conditioner or natural oils to the relaxer.

These treatments also use strong chemicals to permanently straighten hair (new growth will be curly) that can be very harsh—and even carcinogenic. Texturizers are relaxers that are designed to be left on for a short period of time to soften rather than straighten the curl pattern.

We recommend you do careful research before considering a chemical treatment. Results can vary dramatically depending on the texture and condition of your hair.

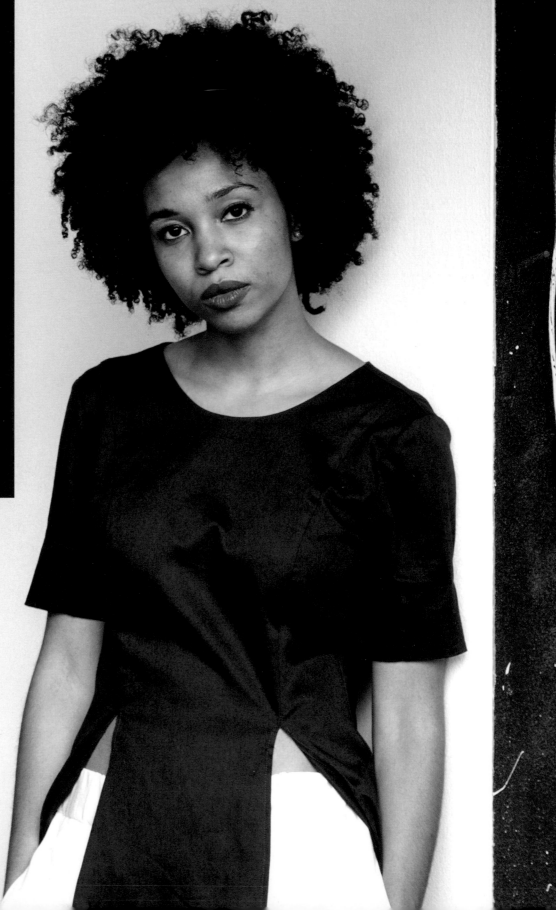

> "The beautiful thing about natural hair is that it's so versatile. I always have many different options to change my hair. It's been a really freeing experience for me."

—Marrisa Wilson, fashion designer

Texture: 3c with some 3b and some 4a, low porosity, coarse, thick

Regimen: I use Hairstory New Wash and Hairstory Hair Balm. If I run out of the Hair Balm, I'll use SheaMoisture Coconut & Hibiscus Curl Enhancing Smoothie.

Chapter 6

GOING NATURAL—

TRANSITIONING, THE BIG CHOP, AND
EVERYTHING IN BETWEEN

After years of relaxing and coloring her hair, Jamila Pope had come to a crossroads. She had significant breakage all over her head. And straight hair, she felt, made her look plain. She scoured social media and discovered a whole world of women who had gone natural.

"There were people doing the Big Chop and letting their hair do its thing," says Pope, who headed to the salon at her local Wal-Mart in 2009 to have a stylist cut off all her relaxer.

After years of having straight, relaxed hair, it took Pope time to get used to her new, unfamiliar texture. She had to discover which styles and products worked best for her 4c coils. Since her Big Chop, she has experimented with a variety of looks, including flat twists and twist outs. Styling her natural hair takes more time than she expected, but she has no regrets.

"Going natural was the healthiest decision I made for my hair, and I never looked back," says Pope.

Many of NaturallyCurly's first and most passionate community members were women who wanted to stop relaxing

> " I love the uniqueness and versatility of curly hair. I can have big curly hair in the morning, and slick smooth hair in the afternoon. I also like how deceiving the length is. It's always a surprise every time I straighten it."

—Sydney Atkinson, financial analyst

Texture: 3c, low porosity, fine, thick

Regimen: I use CURLS Blueberry Bliss Twist N Shout Cream with Eco Styler Krystal Styling Gel.

their hair. Going natural was a relatively new phenomenon in 1998, with few places to turn to for advice. This growing acceptance and celebration of natural hair was a huge driver of the Curl Revolution.

In those early days, many of these women were the first in their families to go natural, and they often faced intense resistance to their decision. One of CurlTalk's busiest threads is still the "Grow-Out Challenge" created by a group of women who wanted to celebrate their progress and get support from each other as they embark on their natural journey.

"October will be my 5th month with no relaxer. I have braids in right now. My goal is to look past the negativity (by my family, of all people)," wrote one CurlTalker on the Grow-Out thread.

"I have some days where I want to relax it just because I'm used to wearing real funky, short haircuts. But whenever I look at my daughters, they give me inspiration and motivation to remain natural," chimed in another.

For most black women, getting a relaxer was a given. "It was a rite of passage," says Veronica Robertson. "You got your hair permed (the term for getting a relaxer) at twelve. That was what you were supposed to do. Or else you used a press and comb in front of the stove or braided it."

Natural hair was considered "bad hair" by many in the black community. Because of this societal pressure, the decision to go natural was, and still is, a difficult, emotional, and daunting one for many women. They have had to face the double whammy of dealing with unsupportive—and sometimes outright hostile—family members and friends, while at the same time learning how to work with an unfamiliar texture they may not have seen since they were young.

There are many reasons why women choose to go natural.

The breakage and hair loss that can be caused by long-term use of relaxers is a major driver. The process of permanently altering the hair's texture leaves the hair shaft weak and vulnerable to damage. Relaxers strip away natural oils and can irritate your scalp. With extended relaxer use, the hair becomes brittle, dry, damaged, and porous, and often breaks off before the desirable length can be achieved. Permanent color or highlights can exacerbate these issues.

For many women, natural hair is a glorious fashion statement. There is plenty of inspiration from other naturalistas—from friends to influencers to celebrities. Natural newbies can look forward to the unfettered flexibility natural hair offers.

"For me, the best part of natural hair is the versatility," says Nasstassia Davy, known as NKNaturals on her social media channels. "I've done twist outs, braid outs, finger coils, flexi-rod sets, perm rod sets, roller sets and more. My go-to style is a twist out, because it's the quickest and easiest style for me."

Davy did her Big Chop in 2012 and regularly posts her styles online. "When I was relaxed, my hair was almost always in a ponytail or a bun. But when I went natural, my curls afforded me the opportunity to be adventurous with my hair and try new things."

For Daniela Gomes, going natural was a political statement. Gomes, an activist in the Brazilian black political movement, said the Afro is a symbol of black power in her country. After relaxing her hair since she was 7-years-old, she decided to go natural in her late twenties.

"In Brazil, an Afro is more than just a hair style," Gomes says. "It's an affirmation. Wearing my hair like this is a statement. It's a way of proving who I am as a black woman."

Curiosity can also be a motivating factor. After getting relaxers since she was six years old, Makaela Chonjontae

Brown-Holt wanted to know what her natural hair looked like.

"I never noticed my hair was being altered with chemicals," Brown-Holt says. "I just thought that *was* my natural hair because it had been getting relaxed for so long. January 2015 was my last relaxer because I wanted to start appreciating my natural tresses."

Whatever drives your desire to go natural, it's easier now than it's ever been. The number of products for natural hair has exploded over the past decade. A growing number of stylists are now skilled at working with curls and coils, and can provide cutting and styling options throughout your journey, whether you decide to do an immediate Big Chop or transition over time. Education and support are readily available—from social media to natural hair events.

Where Do You Start?

Because you've been styling straightened hair, you may be unsure about how to manage your natural texture. That's okay. Try not to get frustrated in the beginning. Nearly everyone who has gone natural will say, "Be patient." As your hair grows in, you'll discover your curl pattern, density, texture, and you'll learn which products and techniques work best

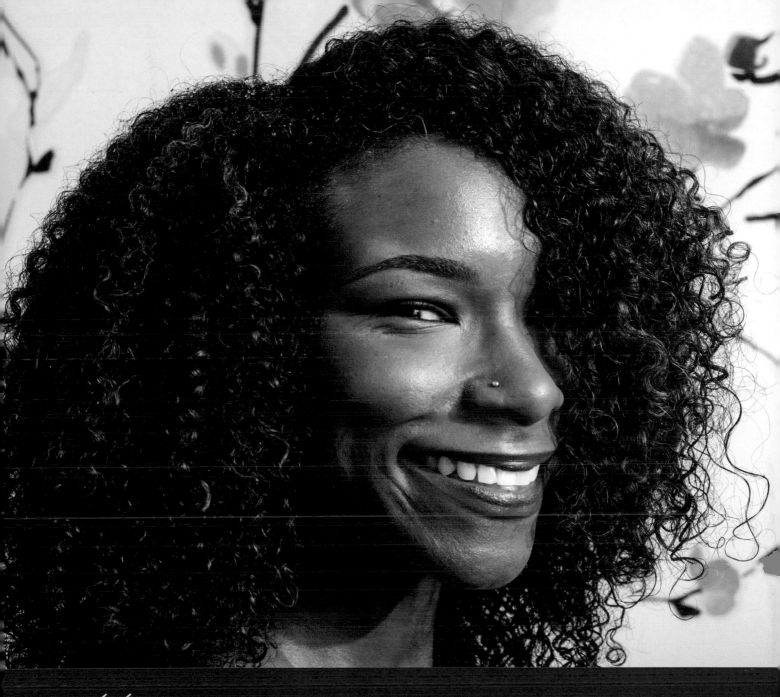

> "I originally went natural in 2004, but I did not know how to maintain it. I ended up getting frustrated so I relaxed my hair. I went natural again in 2012. There were more resources and I had friends to encourage me and teach me."

—Natasha Nash, teacher

Texture: 3c, high porosity, coarse, thick

Regimen: I cleanse once a week with Trader Joe's Tea Tree Shampoo and Conditioner, CURLS Blueberry Bliss Reparative Leave-in conditioner. I rake CURLS Blueberry Bliss Reparative Curl Control Jelly through my hair and sit under a dyer.

"I fried it so much with flat irons. It had terrible heat damage. I killed it. Every time I got a relaxer, I had quarter-sized burns in my scalp. I talked about going natural. One day after work, I looked at my line of demarcation. I got out a spray bottle and started cutting and cutting until I had an inch of hair, and I cried. I took a picture of my now-husband as he came through the door."

—Tauri Laws-Phillips, improv comic, VP of marketing for American English Hair

Texture: 4a, high porosity, fine, thin

Regimen: I use the L.O.C. Method with Macadamia Ultra Moisturizing Conditioner and Masque, Garren Ever Oil, American English Multi-Vitamin Nourishing Spray.

> " I love my curls, even though they can be very frustrating at times. My curls definitely have their own personality. My favorite look is when my hair is down and it's big and has tons of volume, with a part on the side."

—Tylur Starks, singer/songwriter

Texture: 3c, low porosity, fine, thick

Regimen: I like Neutrlab Cocoa Curl Cleansing Conditioner and Neutrlab Pop Curls. I deep condition with that under a hooded dryer.

for your hair. Most naturalistas have been tempted at least once to go back to relaxing.

Saying good-bye to relaxers requires a different mindset and a newfound confidence. You'll have to learn to embrace and love your natural texture, and that can take time. You'll also need to prepare yourself for the world's reaction to your hair—both positive and negative.

"All of a sudden you realize 'Oh, my God. This is me. This is what I look like.' This is how I was made, and it's good enough," says curl expert Anthony Dickey. "I can be fly and contemporary and have all these different looks that I couldn't have when my hair was relaxed because of the limitations."

Realize that you're not alone. There's a whole world of women out there that have made the same decision and have come out on the other side loving their natural texture. The great thing is that there's no right or wrong way to do it.

You can "transition," the process of gradually growing out your relaxer. Or you can do it all at once by doing a "Big Chop"—cutting all your relaxed hair off early in the process in order to go natural right away. Your decision should be based on your lifestyle and your willingness to make a dramatic change.

Transitioning: Take It Slowly

The most gradual approach is called transitioning. As your natural, healthy, and textured hair grows out, you stop applying relaxing chemicals. You simply let it grow. Some curlies find this method to be the ideal solution because they don't have to cut their hair short and can adjust slowly to their natural curls.

It may feel like your hair has a split personality when you are transitioning because, well, that's because it basically does. You will have to manage two completely different textures at the same time.

There's the new growth at your roots, which may be dry and frizzy. Then there are the processed ends, which may be brittle and highly delicate. Your new curls will need the addition of lots of moisture to stay soft and healthy, so it's important to find a moisturizing cleansing conditioner or sulfate-free shampoo that won't dry out your hair. Many successful long-term transitioners sacrifice frequent styling for length retention.

You'll have a line of demarcation—the point at which your relaxed and natural hair meet. Your hair will be especially weak in this section.

You should expect a lot of shedding and breakage because you are cutting the hair

> " In Brazil, there is resistance to natural hair. Brazil is a mostly black country, but it tries to deny anything related to blackness. Hair like mine—Afro hair—is called bad hair. If you wear your natural hair, they ask why are you are letting this black hair come out of your head."

—Daniela Gomes, Brazilian journalist and activist

Texture: 4a/4b/4c, low porosity, fine, thick

Regimen: I use SheaMoisture Superfruit Complex 10-in-1 Renewal Masque and Cantu Shea Butter Coconut Curling Cream.

> "I woke up one morning and was tired of relaxing. I began cutting it off. I had never really seen my face open. It was a shock. It took a while to like what I had going on. I had to relearn myself—how to feel confident walking out of the house with curly hair. I had to relearn how to feel beautiful without it long and flowy."

—Storm Tyler, professor of digital media

Texture: 4a, high porosity, fine, medium density

Regimen: I use Aussie Super Moist Conditioner, Kinky-Curly Knot Today Leave-in Conditioner and Eco Styler Olive Oil Styling Gel.

off from the chemical you've been giving it for a long time," says celebrity natural hairstylist and international beauty speaker Felicia Leatherwood. "So, essentially the hair will begin to rebel."

For clients who want to transition, "I will advise that we look at some hairstyles together online to discover a style that suits them and their lifestyle," Leatherwood says.

The transitioning process can take up to two years, and each stage may present its own unique set of challenges—and opportunities. The products and styles you choose may change over time. You will want to reduce the amount of heat styling and make sure your hair gets the moisture it needs.

"You want to make sure the new hair coming in stays soft and doesn't get dried out, and also that the relaxed hair doesn't get any more damage than it has," Dickey says.

Plan to see your stylist every four to six weeks; you will need to commit to regular trims to gradually get rid of the damaged straight ends.

One option transitioners turn to is called "protective styling." These protective styles—braids, twists, and Bantu knots are some popular options—serve two purposes. They make the hair look good and they also minimize style damage while your curls grow out. Some transitioners opt for extensions and weaves, keeping in mind that these styles shouldn't be installed too tightly or left in too long because they can break the hair. It's also important to remove them every

Upswept into a pompadour, accented with pearls.

" I don't like locs. I love locs! I love the endless styling possibilities— the fact that you can take something that can, at times, look unkempt and come up with the most sophisticated, artistic-looking hair style."

—Maria Thompson, specialist in locs, twists and other natural hair styles

Texture: Locs

Regimen: I wash and do hot-oil treatments for conditioning. Go light on products and stay away from anything that's rich and creamy because it builds up. Keep it simple.

> " I used to perm my hair.
> I had the best perm
> I ever had, but it made me
> realize that I didn't want to
> perm my hair anymore. I
> didn't like the way it felt. I'm
> now fully natural. I feel bold-
> er—a rebel with a cause. My
> hair is a political statement."

**—Angelica Cruz, college
student, rugby player**

Texture: 3c, high porosity,
fine, thick

Regimen: I pre-moisturize so
it's not so heavy with TGIN
Butter Cream Daily Moisturizer.
I don't shampoo, I condition.

three to four weeks to give the scalp a chance to rest. "Anything longer than that will damage the hair and becomes unhygienic for the scalp," says Dickey.

And some transitioners find that wigs can help them through the process, especially with the huge selection of options available in a variety of textures and colors. Full and half wigs, usually accompanied with either a drawstring or wig clips, are quick and easy to install. U-part wigs allow for more natural hair to be exposed, which makes for better blending.

The Big Chop: A Fresh Start

Many women choose an immediate Big Chop. This is when a person, very early in the transitioning process, cuts off all her relaxed hair at once. This is a good solution for those who are ready for a big change immediately, and want to rid themselves of chemically treated hair right away.

You can do the Big Chop anytime—six weeks or six months or two years after your last relaxer. When you decide to get the cut is very personal. Some women do it as soon as they decide to go natural because their hair is very damaged or because they want to embrace change right away, while some women prefer to grow out their hair

to a particular length to avoid a super-short cut. Others sometimes get fed up with dealing with two different textures and take the plunge during the transitioning process. Some call this a "Mini Chop"—waiting until their hair is a little longer before cutting the chemically treated strands off.

Most experts agree that the phrase "Big Chop" is less about at what point in the going-natural process you cut your relaxed hair, and more about how it makes you feel. Regardless of how long your natural hair is, cutting off your relaxed ends is an emotional moment—one that signifies a meaningful point in your journey to naturalness.

"I recently Big Chopped because of all the damage," says Myleik Teele. Teele had Big Chopped several times, but this one was especially traumatic. To get it even, she had to get a buzz cut.

"I was sad, devastated," Teele says. "I knew I'd have a long way to go before I could have any hair to play with. After a week of compliments, I got over it."

If you do the Big Chop early in your journey, you may have a TWA (teeny weeny Afro), ear-length curls, or a tight fade. Whatever your style, you will need to learn to care for your natural hair and figure out which products work best for your hair. This will

> " I'm two years natu-
> ral. I wanted a fresh
> start. I feel like I'm true to
> myself. Before, I wore a lot
> of weaves with perms. I was
> covering up. Now I don't
> have to hide."

**—Tiffany Lopez-Mays, creator
of Oh Tiff! vegan nail polish**

Texture: 3c, low porosity,
fine, thick

Regimen: I use ORS Black
Olive Oil Repair 7 Leave-in
Treatment and ORS Black
Olive Oil Repair 7 Oil Elixir. I
put my fingers through my
hair in the shower and comb
out the tangles.

"I feel like I'm more confident in my natural look. I don't wear makeup on a daily basis. I feel liberated and free to be myself."

—Shellyann Honeghan, nurse and graduate student in social work

Texture: 4c, low porosity, fine, thick

Regimen: I co-wash once a week with Suave Conditioner from the dollar store. I use SheaMoisture Jamaican Black Castor Oil Strengthen, Restore & Grow Shampoo, Jamaican Black Castor Oil Strengthen, Restore & Grow Leave-in Conditioner, and grape seed oil.

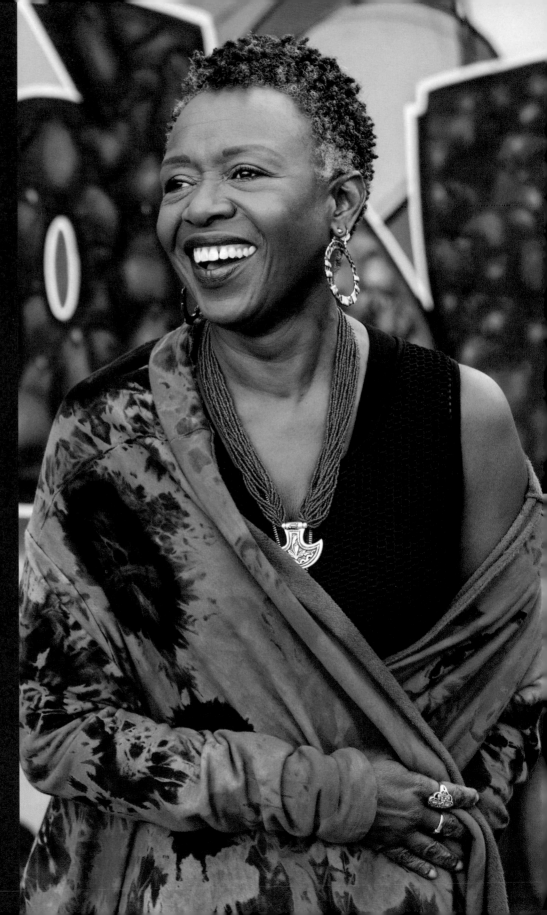

> "I didn't choose natural hair. Natural hair chose me. My hair was always breaking with relaxers. I was never happy with the results. When I was 19, I stopped relaxing my hair. All through college, I wore my hair natural. I was able to create a successful salon based on my own natural hair journey."

—Diane Bailey, stylist/educator, industry leader, advocate, author

Texture: 3c-4b, medium porosity, coarse, thick

Regimen: SheaMoisture has been my "go to" for more than five years. In the winter months, to protect my hair from the cold outdoors and the dry heat indoors, I use the L.O.C. method daily to rehydrate my hair using SheaMoisture Jamaican Black Castor Oil Strengthen, Grow & Restore Collection, and the Coconut Hibiscus Curl Enhancing Smoothie. In the warm summer months, I prefer to use a lighter option by making my own "cocktail" for daily hydration. In a spray bottle, I use 3 oz. water, 10 drops of SheaMoisture Raw Shea Butter Finishing Elixir and 1 oz. of SheaMoisture Omega 3, 6, 9 Rescue + Repair Conditioner. My cocktail has a milky consistency and I use it daily to rehydrate my coils.

take some experimenting, but luckily, your shorter length will make the process easier and less time-consuming.

Your texture will continue to evolve as your natural curls grow. You will want to continue to educate yourself throughout every phase.

It's not uncommon for the hair to get thicker as it gets longer, says Miko Branch, cofounder of Miss Jessie's, a line of hair care products. "As the hair starts growing and changing, you are going to have to grow and change, too, as you learn how to manage it."

Many naturalistas wonder why they waited so long.

"It's so simple and light and free," says Tina Harmon, a stay-at-home mother, who went natural three years ago and is now wearing locs. "Just go for it. Enjoy the process!"

TIPS FOR SURVIVING—AND SAVORING—YOUR BIG CHOP

It may not be the right decision for everyone, but doing the Big Chop can be one of the most transcendent moments you'll experience during your journey to natural hair. Here are some Big Chop tips from NaturallyCurly experts and community members.

Just Do It!

If you are weighed down with doubt, don't make a decision you'll regret, but know that it's just hair and it *will* grow back. There's something about the Big Chop that makes you *own* your natural! If you've made the decision to go natural, there's nothing to it but to just do it!

Be Mentally Prepared

The Big Chop is the first step of a wonderful journey, and it's best to have your head fully in the game before your cut. Think thoroughly not only about the cut itself, but also about what lies beyond. What are the ramifications—in all aspects of your life—of going natural? This is a significant personal decision that you have to be sure you're ready for. Ask your friends, your stylist, and other curlies about their experiences and for any advice they'd give to someone contemplating a Big Chop.

Share Your Plans

You may also want to inform your spouse, family, and friends of your plan, not just so they feel included in your decision, but also

Iyore Moelle Olaye hasn't seen her natural texture since she was 6 years old, when her hair was first relaxed for Easter. She continued relaxing and wearing extensions through high school, college, and her first corporate job as an engineer.

"I wasn't really able to bring my natural self in to work, given the reality of those environments and the level of inclusiveness," Olaye says.

In her current job as a product engineer at Walker & Co., which makes health and beauty solutions for people of color, it seemed like an ideal time for her to go natural. "I'm very interested in learning about who I am and growing as a professional. And it starts with my hair. This is a new beginning."

As she sits in the chair at the Hair Rules Salon in New York—with stylist Anthony Dickey about to cut off her extensions and reveal her new natural growth—she's nervous and scared. She isn't sure what to expect. "I'm stepping into the unknown. I hope I'll be able to embrace it. I'm worried about whether I'll be able to pull it off."

The process takes several hours, as Dickey and his team carefully remove her weave and cut away all of her relaxed hair; several inches fall to the floor. Then he carefully shapes it in a new style that will work well with her new natural texture.

Three weeks later, Olaye loves her 4a hair. It wasn't necessarily love at first sight. "The first week was rough," she says. "One day I woke up and my hair looked like a straw hat."

Once she figured out the products that worked best and the right way to apply them, she has watched with delight as her curls and coils have popped up. She has been trying different styles and is loving twist outs.

"It is much easier to manage than I ever imagined. I spend less time daily maintaining my styles than I did with my extensions and relaxed hair. I am still adjusting to the styles I like best. I am excited to continue on the journey."

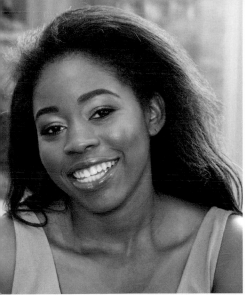
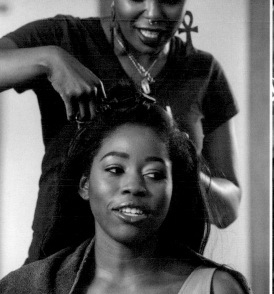
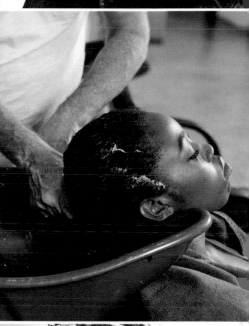
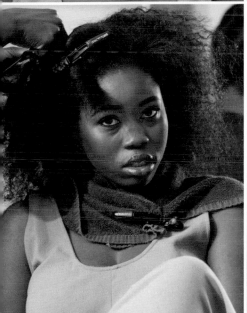
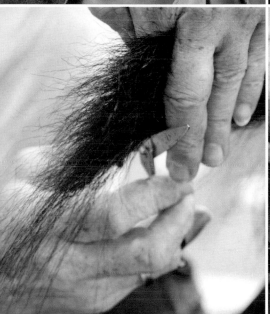
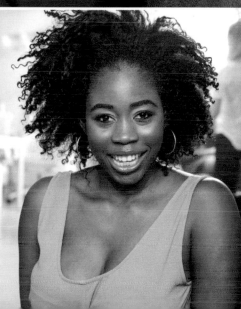
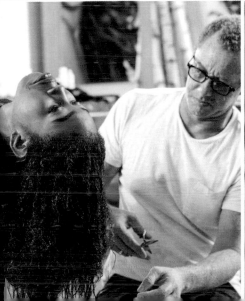
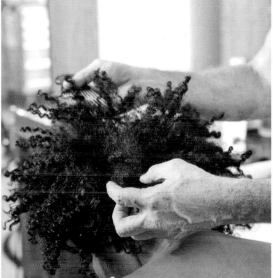

to gauge their reactions, positive or otherwise. Don't be discouraged by any negative reactions; just remember that you're doing this for you.

Plan Ahead

You should also prepare your regimen before doing the Big Chop so you aren't overwhelmed. You won't have a whole bunch of hair to work with once you Big Chop, so your routine and the products you use will be very important. Research the brands, products, and ingredients you may want to try after you Big Chop.

Keep It Simple

As you're planning, keep simplicity in mind. After you do it, you may be in a fragile state of mind and an easy-care routine will give you one less thing to worry about. Whether you have half an inch or a few inches of hair after your cut, the best thing you can do is to keep things simple with your routine and product use.

Be Patient

Give your products an opportunity to see if they will work by using each one consistently for a few weeks.

Enjoy It!

You might be surprised at how quickly the TWA stage goes by, so be sure to embrace and enjoy this new style and your new self! The TWA and the subsequent grow-out phase offer a fantastic opportunity to play around with inventive new styles. Have fun with your beautiful new natural hair—and pat yourself on the back for having had the courage to do it!

Go online to check out how-to videos and style pics.

HOW TO STYLE TRANSITIONING HAIR

Styling can present challenges and opportunities during transitioning. If you thought styling one texture was hard, try working with two at the same time! Remember, your goal is to keep the new growth as healthy as possible, so you'll want to use styling techniques that blend your two textures without creating any more damage. Many experts (and curlies

#curl**talk**

ADVICE FROM OUR COMMUNITY ABOUT TRANSITIONING

"If you're transitioning or thinking about it, just know it's a long road. But there's a lot of information out there now to help."

"Don't go crazy over buying hair products. Give your hair time to adjust to the new products and make time to learn your hair, practice protective styling, and enjoy the journey!"

"Transition the way that fits your personality, your lifestyle, so if it's Big Chop or slow, don't beat yourself up, PERIOD."

"Prayer is key, 'cause it does require a lot of patience. You can choose to do it long term, but it will grow faster once the straight ends are off. Don't listen to the negativity. Embrace you!"

"Don't compare your hair to someone who's worn theirs natural all their life; theirs won't be as frizzy because they didn't go through what you did!"

"Don't give up, and know it will be worth it once you have your hair completely transitioned. My hair is healthier and much easier to maintain. It's awesome!"

" My favorite look is definitely a twist out. It's easy to maintain and gives me the volume I want every time. Being natural is work, but in the end it's worth it. My hair has never been so healthy!"

—Kay Price, caseworker for the Texas Department of Health & Human Services

Texture: 4b/4c, high porosity, coarse, thick

Regimen: I pre-'poo with coconut oil, shampoo and condition with the Shea Moisture Jamaican Black Castor Oil collection. For stylers I use Eco Styler Gel and SheaMoisture Coconut & Hibiscus Curl Enhancing Smoothie. I always sleep with a satin bonnet and do 10-minute scalp massages with castor oil every other day.

> "My favorite look is the 'frohawk'—a mohawk with an Afro appearance. It's easy to style and can complement any attire, whether formal or casual. All I do is pin up each side, fluff the front, middle, and back, and that's it!"

—Candice Johnson, Quality Assurance

Texture: 3c, low porosity hair, fine, medium density

Regimen: I cowash (with regular Suave conditioner mixed with olive oil). I always spray my hair with water before applying any products. My go-to products are Kinky-Curly Knot Today Leave-In Conditioner Detangler, Kinky-Curly Curling Custard, Nature's Way Extra Virgin Coconut Oil, and Let's Jam! Shining and Conditioning Gel (for my edges).

> "I've been wearing my braid extensions for a while. It takes three hours and costs $15 to buy the hair. I don't have to do my hair every day. It prevents heat damage and it makes my hair grow. Everyone really loves it. They ask how I did it and how long it took. They want their hair done like it."

—Courtney Crook, stylist

Texture: 4c, high porosity, fine, thick

Regimen: I wake up, put mousse on my hair, a little bit of oil and I'm good for the day.

in the know) recommend protective styles—low-manipulation styles that last a few days or longer and don't require much handling, heat, or touch-ups. Here are the top styles for transitioning strands:

Braids

Braids can be individual plaits that fall down loosely. Or, they can be sections of hair gathered together, laying closely against the scalp with no room for movement. Both types of braids effectively hide your ends from potentially harmful effects of regular styling, manipulation, friction against your clothing, and the environment. Popular types of braids include Marley, micro and cornrows.

Box Braids

A type of braided extensions, also referred to as box braids, are another versatile protective style that can last for several weeks if properly cared for.

Heat-Free Curls

Hair rollers help you get voluminous, uniform, long-lasting curls and waves without an iron or wand, and there are many options for every budget and skill level. Perm rods are easy to use and come in many sizes, so they are good for short to long hair. Many curlies like the ease of flexi rods, which are bendable, cushioned, and affordable.

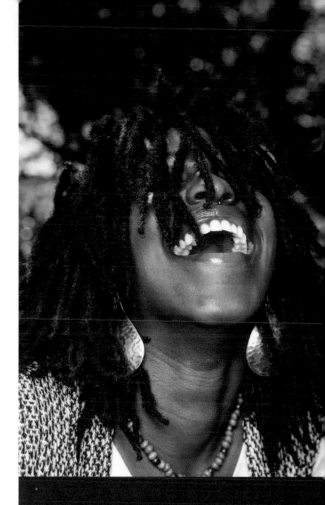

" My mother had done my hair my whole life. I had to learn what to do with this new entity on my head. The possibilities were endless."

—Kayla Ann McLeod, yoga instructor, food server

Texture: Locs

Regimen: I mix some rosemary oil, water, and a little bit of lavender—sometimes eucalyptus—in a spray bottle. I spritz it in and work through some sort of moisturizer. I product hop.

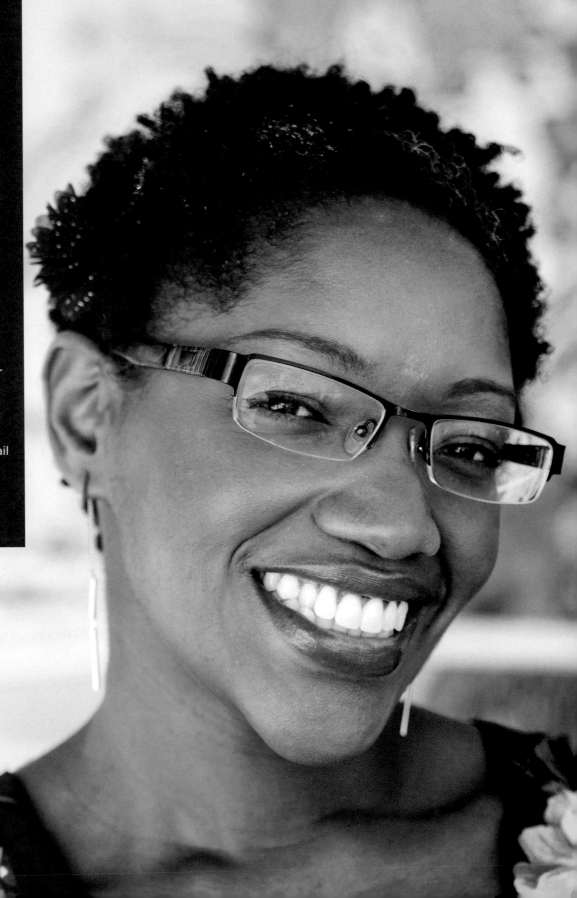

> " I didn't know it was called 'going natural.' My mom went natural and didn't have to worry about heat damage or keeping it straight. It seemed easier than forcing my hair into a style that's not natural."
>
> **—Cynthia Sullivan, academic counselor**

Texture: 4b, low porosity, coarse, thick

Regimen: I deep condition my hair once or twice a week with ORS Olive Oil Replenishing Pak Deep Penetrating Conditioner. I wash with shampoo once a week and co-wash every two to three weeks with Mane n' Tail Original Conditioner.

Locs

This hairstyle, also known as dreadlocks or dreads, is ropelike strands of hair formed by matting or braiding the hair. Locs come in many different forms. They can be curled, braided, pinned up, cut into a style and colored. If you're thinking about locs, you may want to consult a loctician.

Turbans, Scarves, and Head Wraps

Turbans and head wraps have been popping up on the fashion radar all over the place. They have been seen as signature pieces on fashion show runways and as bold accessories on the red carpet.

Twists

Many of these styles use a two-strand braiding technique that, like some braided styles, allows the hair to be separated in freeform sections that have the freedom of movement. Twists are versatile enough to be combined and pinned up, also qualifying them as updos (the third type of protective style). There are a wide range of twists, from 2-strand to flat twists.

Updos

A hairstyle that calls for your hair to be tucked away, smoothed down, and held away from your face is known as an updo. Updos can range from a high bun to a top knot.

Bantu Knots

Named after sub-Saharan Africa's far-migrating Bantu peoples, Bantu knots look like tightly coiled little knots of hair. They're created when sections of hair are twisted and pinned into place. Transitioners can wear the knots for a couple days or more, then unpin the knots to reveal uniform waves and curls, and voilà!—yet another hairstyle.

Wigs

If you'd rather give your entire head a break from manipulation and styling, opt for a wig, which allows the hair to rest.

Extensions

Hair extensions allow you to go from curly to wavy, wavy to curly, and from long to short. You can even get bangs, without having to wait for your hair to grow.

"I do yarn braids. I've been wearing them on and off for four years. I get bored so easily with everything—especially hair color. I go to Michael's because they have a huge selection of yarn. I can only use 100% acrylic because other kinds of strands can rip the hair out. I've been gray, blue, black, and white. Now I'm wearing calico."

—Erin Kamile Jean Walker, server, vocalist, and music engineer

Texture: 4c, medium porosity, coarse, thick

Regimen: I use water, jojoba oil and tea tree oil in a spray bottle.

> " My go-to style is the ninja bun. If my hair is braided, I take the braids out and fluff my hair. Then I take a portion of the front—based on how big I want it to be—and pull my hair out. I get gel and a bristle brush and brush the top of my head. Then I tie it up, and use bobby pins to get the bun look. I discovered it by accident. One day I had a great twist out, and I wanted it to be half up and half out. I thought maybe I'll try the ninja bun and now it's my go-to look."

—Erica Patterson, pre-K teacher

Texture: 4c, medium porosity, coarse, thick

Regimen: I co-wash every two weeks with Garnier Whole Blends Avocado Oil & Shea Butter Nourishing Conditioner. I also use coconut oil and Cantu Shea Butter Leave-in Conditioner.

> " Mona from Muze Salon opened my eyes. She helped me to embrace frizz and big hair. That's been my mission: What you have is yours and you should embrace it."

—Hortensia Caires, photographer, influencer, creator of StyleFeen social media platform

Texture: 3b/3c, low porosity, coarse, thick

Regimen: Once a week, I wash with Kinky-Curly Come Clean Shampoo and Kinky-Curly Knot Today Leave-in Conditioner. I also use Eden Body Coconut Shea Cleansing Cowash, DevaCurl SuperCream Coconut Curl Styling Cream, and Bounce Curl Light Crème Gel With Aloe.

Chapter 7

CUTTING CURLS—

UNLOCKING THE POTENTIAL OF YOUR TEXTURE

Can a good haircut change your entire outlook on life?

> "Wow! After so many bad haircuts I just decided to spend the money and go to a curly hair professional and my results were great! Nice and layered. My hair overall had more volume, style, and shape! Bye-bye triangle—the cut is worth every penny!"
>
> "I am *finally* in love with my long, curly hair. He gave me the best haircut I've ever had and took the time to listen to what I wanted."

The short answer is yes, as these NaturallyCurly stylist reviews show. You can't describe the confidence that comes when you get a great haircut. It doesn't matter whether it's a light dusting—a term for the tiniest of trims—or a dramatic change. When the cut is good, it can change your life.

"It wasn't until I got a good cut for curly hair that I really loved my hair," says blogger Hortensia Caires, known online as StyleFeen.

Why is a haircut so powerful? For starters, a good curly cut will make your hair look and feel healthier. It will work with your texture and your lifestyle, arming you with the skills to maintain the look. It can also dramatically cut down on styling time. The right shape will complement your features.

A great curly cut can entirely change the way you view your hair—from seeing it as a flaw to considering it one of your best features—if not your very best feature.

Of course, what we just described is the best-case scenario. Maybe you can't remember a time when you left a salon feeling good about your hair, let alone experiencing a transformative haircut. Many of you probably have had at least one traumatic salon experience, complete with a clueless and/or rude stylist who doesn't understand curly hair, doesn't like working with texture, or immediately steers you to chemical treatments or a blowout. Many stylists don't understand that cutting curly and coily hair is *very* different from cutting straight hair, requiring completely different techniques and training.

"I can cut straight hair with my eyes closed," jokes Christo, global artistic director of Christo Fifth Avenue Salon in New York City and creator of the Curlisto line of hair products.

Why is it so different?

"When cutting curly hair, it is important that I avoid precision, tension, and accuracy—which is the polar opposite to what I do when I'm working with straight hair," says Jonathan Torch. "Curly hair is all about movement and bounce, which are both things that are hard to control—I work with it, not against it."

Believe it or not, textured hair isn't covered in the curriculum in cosmetology school. Most stylists graduate without ever having worked on a curly head. "The word curly and kinky isn't in any textbook in the US," says curl expert Anthony Dickey.

So it's not surprising that so many curlies have had horrible experiences in the styling chair, as these CurlTalk posts illustrate:

> **"I am so mad! It's been almost 2 weeks and at least I'm not crying anymore. No two pieces of hair on my head are the same length. I thought I was very clear about what I wanted. I have one big divot in the side that is hard to disguise but better. My hair takes forever to grow. This is going to take a long time."**

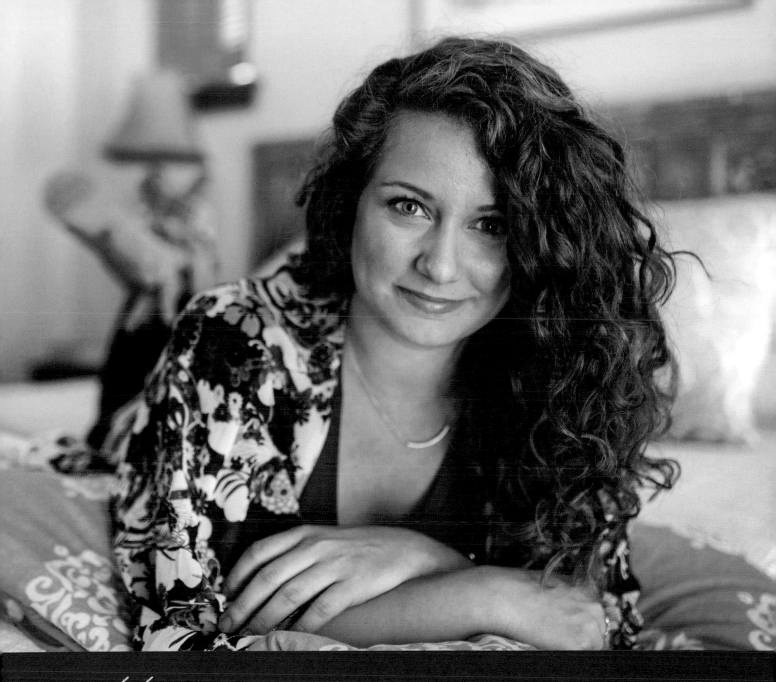

" You have to go to someone who knows curls. I remember looking for stylists. I would ask for someone who was good for curly hair. NaturallyCurly was my resource."

—Maranda Moody, glorified paralegal

Texture: 2c/3a, low porosity, coarse, thick

Regimen: I cleanse with Jason's Sulfate-Free Tea Tree Oil Shampoo twice a week and follow with TRESemmé Naturals Nourishing Moisture Conditioner. I scrunch TRESemmé Mega Hold Sculpting Gel and a little bit of TRESemmé Naturals Nourishing Moisture Conditioner, then tie my hair up in a T-shirt for a few minutes and let it dry overnight. In the morning, I'll occasionally diffuse for extra volume.

> "Stylists in beauty school don't get trained to work with texture. Beauty schools should train you to work with straight-haired clients as well as curly-haired. It should be mandatory. It's our professional responsibility."

—Jane Carter, stylist and founder of Jane Carter Solution

Texture: 3b/3c, high porosity, fine, thick

Regimen: I rinse my hair every day with Jane Carter Solution Nutrient Replenishing Conditioner. I've been playing with Jane Carter Solution Curls to Go Gel.

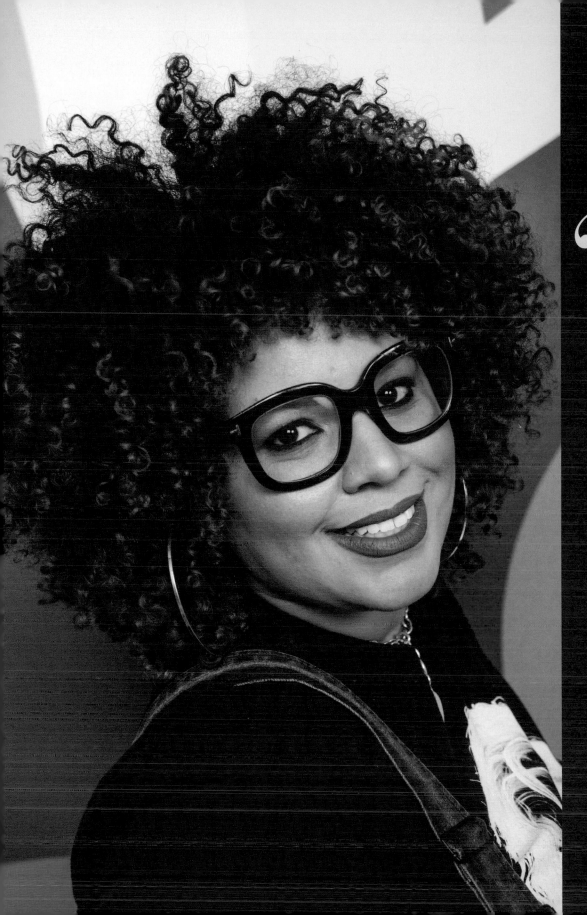

> **"** I made it my mission to impact the industry by exposing salon professionals to what a curly girl *is* and not what a curly girl should be from everyone else's point of view."

—Isabella Vazquez, editorial stylist and founder of Curlpopnhair.com and *curlpopworld*

Texture: 3c, high porosity, fine, thick

Regimen: I wash with Pureology Hydrate Shampoo and clarify once a week with Redken Hair Cleansing Cream Shampoo. I also use Sheamoisture Jamaican Black Castor Oil Strengthen & Grow Leave-in Conditioner, Bounce Curl Light Crème Gel with Aloe, Redken All Soft Argan Multi-6 Multi-Care Oil, and Tigi S-Factor Serious Deep Conditioner.

Christo of Christo Fifth Avenue Salon consults with Mary Tamborra before ever picking up the scissors.

> "So I've just come back from yet another unfortunate hairdresser experience. I tried to be brave. But now that I washed my hair again, I feel like crying. She showed me the length she wanted to cut off and I should have stopped her there. She then chopped off some hair, layered it, and then took out a razor. My hair is less defined, less curly, more frizzy, poufy—just a mess."

But one of the best things about the Curl Revolution is what's happening in salons, behind the chair, where a growing number of stylists are now passionately embracing curls, coils, and waves. Many have taken it upon themselves to get special training at places like the DevaCurl Academy, Christo Fifth Avenue, and Ouidad, or with groups like Curly Hair Artistry so they can master the techniques for working with curls and coils. More salons than ever have dedicated themselves to texture—salons such as Southern Curl in Atlanta and Curls Gone Wild in Gilbert, Arizona, places like Got Curls in Lexington, Kentucky, and Curls on Top in Laguna Beach, California. More than 130 salons in NaturallyCurly's Salon Finder now include the word "Curl" in their title.

Check out NaturallyCurly.com's Salon Finder

The First Step: A Consultation

Any good curl cut should start with a thorough consultation. It's a chance to tell your stylist everything he or she needs to know about your hair—how much it shrinks, how you like to wear it, what has worked in the past and what hasn't.

What's your goal? Are you cutting to maintain a particular shape? Or are you trying to gain length and only want to cut minimal amount to remove damage and split ends? You may not be able to reach your goal in just one haircut.

Shari Harbinger, cofounder of DevaCurl Academy, calls the combined intuitive and technical approach to cutting "psycurlogy." Harbinger, who has been an integral part of DevaCurl since its start, says psycurlogy means getting inside the client's thought process—"where she's been, where she is now, where she wants to go, and what's possible. Our goal is always to reach a mutually shared vision."

You can make the stylist's job easier if you

come to the consultation prepared. He or she needs to see your curls in action—the way they look every day —so don't show up in ponytail or with a blowout if you don't normally wear it straight. Remember that words get lost in translation, especially at the salon, so always bring pictures showing cuts and styles you like to make sure you both are on the same page.

"While the cut [in the photos you bring] might not fit your face structure exactly, it will definitely show the stylist the shape you are looking for and offer a framework to work with," says Diane Da Costa, author of *Textured Tresses*.

Curly girl and NaturallyCurly community member Junysia Jones says she has learned to be very specific with stylists, asking a lot of questions. "Haircuts are scary, and unlike some other services, they're permanent! If your stylist seems irritated with you wanting to ask questions, I'd leave! Any good stylist who's confident in their abilities will not have a problem answering your questions and will explain everything to you to alleviate your concerns."

SO WHAT'S THE BEST WAY TO CUT CURLS?

There is no one best way to cut hair. There are a number of different techniques being used by talented stylists who specialize in curly hair. Each has its own advantages.

Two of the most popular curl-cutting techniques—developed by the curly salons Ouidad and Devachan—essentially have two different schools of thought. DevaCurl believes curls should be cut dry, while Ouidad—who calls her trademarked cutting style the "Carve & Slice"—believes the hair must be wet to get a good cut. There are also many curly stylists and salon owners with years of experience who use a combination of the two, or have developed their own unique cutting style—with fabulous results and a loyal curly clientele.

So which is right for you? Learning about your options is a good place to start, and finding the perfect method for your curls may take some trial and error.

Ultimately, it's important to remember that any good cut should consider the big picture—your curl texture and density, flat spots, the shape of your head, the health of your hair and your style preferences. If you like the option to straighten your hair, you may choose a different cut than someone who always wears her hair in its natural texture.

"When I got my first dry cut, I was used to wearing it curly," recalls CurlTalker Angeluv. "I loved it when my hair was curly. But when I straightened it the next day, it was uneven."

Cutting Dry

The dry cut, known by some as the "Deva Cut," is a technique made famous by Lorraine Massey and the stylists at the Devachan Salon in New York City. The logic: cutting curls in their dry state allows the stylist to better see the way your hair curls naturally—their shape and their spring   and gives more control over shaping the hair. Each ringlet is trimmed individually, as needed. (Remember, curls appear longer when they are wet but shrink back up as they dry.) The stylist sculpts a haircut to your head, individually trimming each ringlet. With the dry cut, it's about where you choose to cut. It's more about shape than length. You end up with a cut that is customized to your natural texture.

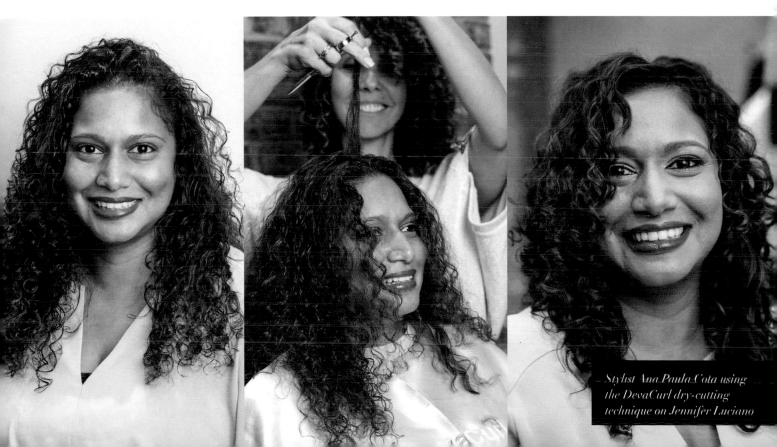

Stylist Ana Paula Cota using the DevaCurl dry-cutting technique on Jennifer Luciano

This dry-cutting technique also helps the stylist see the client's "spring factor"—the hair's ability to expand and contract. Stylists who cut the hair dry say it's difficult to predict shrinkage on wet hair. Cutting a quarter inch when the hair is wet can look like an inch when the hair is dry.

"Nobody has an even pattern—they have 2, 3, 4 textures," says Ana Paula Cota, a senior stylist at the Devachan Salon in New York, which has two academies to train stylists in how to work with curly hair. "Cutting it dry, you have a clear vision of what the texture is communicating. You can think about how it's going to grow. Dry cutting works with every texture type."

Cutting Wet

Many curly stylists prefer to work with the method of cutting wet hair. Cutting wet hair is considered the most accurate approach, as the shape of dry curls can morph depending on the day. Ouidad's Carve & Slice technique is performed on wet, freshly cleansed and conditioned hair, much like a straight-hair cut. The difference, however, is that the stylist must consider your spring factor, or he or she could end up cutting too much. An experienced stylist will automatically know how to make these adjustments, whereas a novice most likely won't.

"I only ever cut curly hair when it's wet," Torch says. "When the hair is wet, stylists are able to manipulate the direction that we want your curls to fall, to shrink, or to loosen. Cutting curly hair wet allows for total control and can be adjusted to avoid the cutting shock which creates unflattering, unwanted steps and ledges in the hair that take ages to grow out."

Combination Wet/Dry

This type of cut borrows from the best of both worlds. It combines the accuracy of a precise wet cut and the reality check of how your curls look in their dry state. This can be helpful for someone with several different curl types, such as when one has tighter textures closer to the head that may be not be obvious with wet hair. For example, curly hair veteran Andre Walker likes to start with a dry cut, creating guidelines to see where he wants to see the curls fall, then goes on to cut the hair wet for a more precise result.

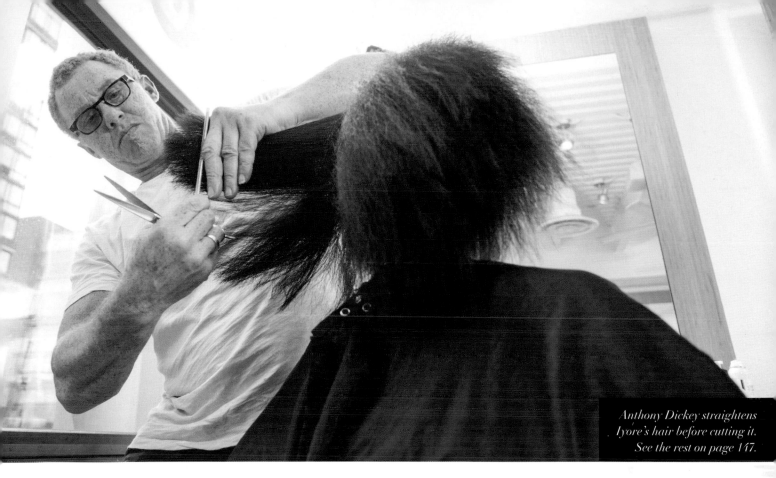

Anthony Dickey straightens
Iyore's hair before cutting it.
See the rest on page 147.

Cutting Straightened Hair

Not to be confused with a styling blowout, sometimes curl stylists will reach for a blow-dryer before the scissors. Don't freak out—this doesn't mean they don't know how to handle textured hair. Certain texture types, like very tight and kinky curls, are easier to cut after they have been straightened into one uniform texture.

"The kinkier or tighter the curl gets, the more I blow it out and cut with it straight," says Dickey, who opts for wet cutting for clients with looser curls or waves.

For tighter textures with a lot of shrinkage, spirals, and tight kinks, he believes blowing it straight enables him to make sure that all strands get the attention they need.

"You can't cut what you can't see," Dickey says. "Just because you have curls, each curl is comprised of hundreds of thousands of strands depending on the thickness of the hair. Often, women with tight curly hair or tight kinky hair have challenges with getting their hair long because they don't get proper haircuts."

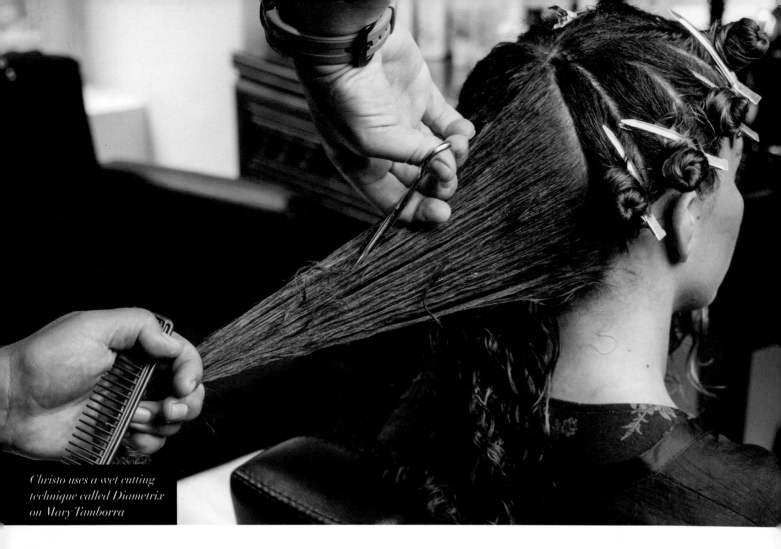

Christo uses a wet cutting technique called Diametrix on Mary Tamborra

SIGNS OF A GOOD STYLIST

There are knowledgeable, trained stylists out there who are passionate about curls, coils, and waves. You just have to know how to find them. Here are good ways to find a curl-savvy stylist.

Another Curly's Recommendation

Word of mouth from other curlies is one of the best ways to find a good stylist. But if you're the only one with your hair type in your family or in your group of friends, don't be discouraged! You can easily access reviews on NaturallyCurly's Salon Finder.

> " I'm still on the journey, getting comfortable with it. It's empowering when you're around other people who understand curly hair. Now I have people who come up and ask what I use."

—Mary Tamborra, research contract manager

Texture: 3b/3c, high porosity, coarse in parts, thick

Regimen: I use DevaCurl One Condition, DevaCurl Coconut Cream Styler, and Bounce Curl Light Crème Gel with Aloe.

And if you see a curly walking down the street with a great haircut, don't be bashful about asking her who cuts her hair

They Ask a Lot of Questions Before Picking up the Scissors

Most good curl stylists will insist on a consultation before they work on your hair. (See main story.) Going in for a consultation before your cut is a good way to ensure that your stylist understands curls, and that she understands *your* curls.

They Know the Curl Lingo

While you're in for your consultation, listen carefully. CG, Plopping, Type 3b. The curly community speaks its own language, and your stylist should know and use that language while discussing your hair. It shows she's been around curlies and, by extension, it shows she understands the needs and challenges of those with curls and coils.

The Salon or Stylist's Instagram Feed (or Portfolio) Is Full of Curls

If there's a salon or stylist in your area that you're interested in trying out, get on their Instagram page or website and take a look at their work. You can see quickly if they are passionate about texture.

They Have Curl Training

Unfortunately, most cosmetology schools still don't train stylists on how to work with texture, which means they can get their license without ever working on a curly head of hair. Luckily, there are a growing number of courses, workshops, and seminars that enable stylists to learn how to work with curls, coils, and waves. Always feel free to ask a stylist about her training, or check her website to see if she has received special training from companies such as DevaCurl, Christo Fifth Avenue, Ouidad, or groups such as Curly Hair Artistry. The best curl stylists are passionate about texture and continually honing their skills.

#curl**talk**

HOW FAR WOULD YOU TRAVEL FOR AN EXPERT CURLY CUT?

Some curly girls, gun-shy from a lifetime of bad haircuts, will travel far and wide to get a haircut from a curl expert. According to our research, curly girls will travel an average of 2 hours to get a good cut. We asked our community how far they've traveled for a haircut, and here is what they told us.

"I took 3 planes to get my haircut in NYC from Australia. I won't let just anyone touch my hair. They also need to be a curl specialist."

"I recently traveled 130 miles from south England to the midlands—Birmingham—it's a long way to go but it's worth it."

"I'm going to have to travel 3 hours to San Francisco to see a loctician. I live in a town with a population of about 91,000+, yet the number of people who even do locs around here I could count on my hand."

"I used to fly three states over to Florida to have a stylist at Ouidad do the Carve & Slice 1–2 times a year."

"I go to get my hair cut with a curly girl-friend 4 times a year. We drive over 3 hours one way, and then head back home—an all-day girl talk, curl talk, life talk. It's cheaper than therapy!"

"My regular hair appointments are now a 2.5-hour drive to Cleveland, Ohio."

"I live in Ireland and the only person I trust to cut my hair is in France. I can only get it cut on holiday."

They're Not Afraid to Say No

There are some things that people with curls cannot or should not do, and a stylist who is experienced with textured hair won't be afraid to tell you. For example, if you have curly hair and bring in a photo of a model with a stick-straight, layered cut, the stylist should let you know that a cut like that would require extreme measures to achieve.

They Make You Feel Good about Your Hair

The best curl stylists will help you see the potential in your hair rather than focusing on the challenges. They focus on the potential of your hair before they start cutting it, even as they're providing advice about how to improve it.

They Teach You How to Do What They Do

How many times have you walked out of the salon with perfect ringlets, but find when you get home, it's impossible to recreate the look? Good curl stylists will teach you their styling techniques—whether teaching you how best to apply product for maximum curl definition, providing tips on diffusing techniques, or demonstrating how to clip your roots to gain height and volume. Some curl salons even host education events for their clients where they demonstrate how to get different looks.

Chapter 8

COLORING CURLS—

A RAINBOW OF OPTIONS

Hazel Marie Stallion's hair color is a big part of her fashion statement, and she's always changing up her look. She used to be platinum blonde, but now rocks a multicolor frohawk. The top is blonde, while the sides are brown. Next, she plans to go back to an all-over black color "until I come across a new color I want to try," she says.

Social media influencer Rhea Carter has made a name for herself with her bold color choices–from cotton candy pink to bright turquoise blue. She colors her hair every three to four months, deciding on her next color based on the season or her mood.

Colorist Stephanie McLemore recently dyed her natural hair from dark brown to honey blonde, with platinum tips. "It completely changed my look," says McLemore, Dark & Lovely's lead style squad member.

"Before I looked like a professor. I felt boring and dull. Now, I have so much more confidence."

One of the most popular and impactful ways to enhance the look of wavy, curly, or coily hair is with color, whether that be all-over color, strategically placed highlights, or trying a popular fantasy color like pink or blue.

But coloring curly hair—because of its porosity, condition, and texture—can be much different from coloring straight hair. You need to take all of these factors into consideration to get the look you want.

Because curls are not a flat surface, they don't reflect the light the way straight hair does. You need to take their curves into consideration, says curl stylist Brianne Prince of Mason, Ohio.

Textured hair is naturally drier and more porous, which may prevent the color from processing into the anticipated shade. Low-porosity hair can deflect light the way it deflects color. High-porosity curls can suck up undertones and pigment and may not deposit evenly on the hair.

For example, a curly girl might see a straight-haired woman with a shade of blonde she really likes but that same shade will appear a shade-and-a-half darker on curly hair, says Isabella Vazquez. "Any time there is a bend, the light reflects differently on it. That's the tricky part when you're a curly girl."

ALL-OVER COLOR: SEMI VS. DEMI VS. PERMANENT

> **"Is it all right to use a semi-permanent over permanent color? I'm not thrilled with my color right now, but I'd kind of like to try out a different color but not commit to permanent."**

Many curlies want to brighten up or change the color of their hair, such as going from blonde to red. While color treatments are fun and exciting, there are different options to choose from based on your specific needs.

Semi- and demi-permanent color is typically a better choice, depending upon how much gray you have, how dramatic you want the color to look, and how long you want your color to last.

Your hair shaft contains three important parts: the medulla, the cortex, and the cuticle. The medulla is the innermost part found in thicker hair types and is often missing from fine hair. The next layer is called the cortex, made up of cells of keratin, which is responsible for 90 percent

> 66 I started dyeing my hair red when *My So-Called Life* was really popular. It started with box color, and then, I started going to a salon. I usually put a professional red rinse on it in-between salon visits to make the color more vibrant."

—Shana Ogg, marketing manager

Texture: 3a/3b, high porosity, fine, medium density

Regimen: I switch between Kevin Murphy's Luxury Wash and Luxury Conditioner and Kerastase Discipline Bain Fluidealiste Shampoo and Conditioner Kerastase Discipline Maskeratine. For styling, I love Kevin Murphy's Motion Lotion Curl Enhancing Lotion and Big Sexy Hair Spray & Play Volumizing Hairspray.

of the strand's weight. It is the cortex that determines the texture and natural color of your hair. The outermost part of the hair is the cuticle, made up of overlapping, colorless cells similar to roof shingles, and it serves as a protective barrier to the cortex.

Demi-permanent color is naturally ammonia-free, has a low pH, and uses a low-volume developer (1:1 ratio) to gently lift the cuticle to penetrate beneath the surface to the cortex, therefore preserving the integrity of the hair. It can cover gray up to 50 percent and can last up to 28 shampoos.

Semi-permanent color adsorbs onto the outside of the hair shaft with some molecules absorbing beneath the cuticle layer, depending on the porosity of the hair. Porous hair will receive more color than non-porous hair. With each shampoo, color is removed and can last up to eight shampoos. Semi-permanents are typically retail products rather than professional and provide up to 30 percent gray coverage.

Want to check out a new trend without a major commitment? Temporary color may be the best choice for you. Compared to permanent color, temporary hair color is a larger molecule that coats the surface of the hair and doesn't penetrate deep into the cuticle. Because harsh chemicals aren't involved in the process, you can switch things up as often as you'd like.

No developer is used and little to no gray coverage is expected. However, when applied to pre-lightened or damaged/porous hair, temporary color may stain the hair shaft. To make your temporary hair color last a bit longer and look a tad brighter, cover with a plastic cap and sit under heated dryer for 30–45 minutes.

If you're looking for a more dramatic change, or if you're looking for significant gray coverage, then you will want to use a single-process permanent color. Depending on your hair and the percentage that's gray, you may need to repeat the coloring process every six to eight weeks.

"If your main goal is to cover gray, permanent color is a must," McLemore says. "Gray hair can be very stubborn."

HIGHLIGHTS

> "I have been wanting to get highlights, but how do they turn out in curly hair? Would my hair get really damaged? Would they even show up? Would it take longer to highlight my hair?"

Many experts in coloring curls have created their own highlighting techniques that provide more control and allow them to highlight individual curls. One such technique is called Pintura, and was developed by Denis da Silva of Devachan Salon. The dye is painted directly onto the strands, enabling the stylist to place highlights strategically and achieve a natural-looking effect.

"Because curly hair lives off the scalp, you are starting with a fabric that has dimension and volume and movement," says Shari Harbinger, cofounder of DevaCurl Academy. "You have to understand the fabric and bring it to life. It's more of a strategic placement of where I want the color to live in order to capture the movement and beauty of the curls and their shape."

Harbinger says she can accent those specific curls not only to bring out the beauty of the cut but to bring them to life, "customizing by choosing selected curl families and curl cluster groups. . . . You are relying both on a creative eye and technical roadmap."

At Ouidad, many stylists use balayage to highlight their clients' curls. Balayage is another painted-on technique that allows the stylist to selectively apply the lightener/color to enhance the natural texture.

Because textured hair lives in motion, a full color from root to end is not necessary to achieve a highlighted look—a strategic mid-shaft application may yield the optimal look.

It is especially important to avoid over-processing textured hair to prevent it from getting

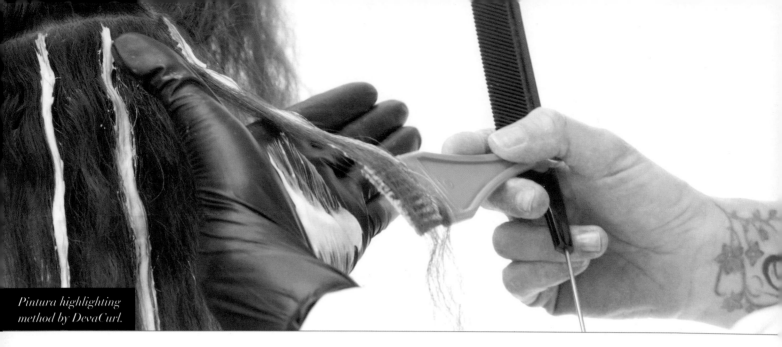

dry and damaged. Over-processed highlights can also make curly hair look frizzier, something many curlies want to avoid.

Another coloring technique that looks especially good on curly hair is ombre. Ombre is the gradual lightening of the hair strand, usually fading from a darker color near the roots to a lighter one at the ends. Ombre can be very subtle or very striking.

HENNA

Because some curlies are hyper-sensitive to moisture and damage, some women have sought a less-damaging alternative to hair dyes. Henna is a popular choice for dyeing the hair because it does not contain harsh ammonia and peroxides. It can even have benefits such as adding thickness and shine.

Henna is able to penetrate the hair and adhere to the strands. The dye deposit fills in the gaps, which is how it is able to strengthen the hair. Depending on how long you leave it on your hair, the ingredients you mix in, and the natural color of your hair, your color will range from deep orange to burgundy or coffee brown.

"Henna works best for those with healthy, porous hair," says henna expert Khadija Dawn Carryl, president and creative director of Henna Sooq, which provides henna, tools, and education. "The henna will then absorb more easily and colors the hair really well."

For those who don't fit this criteria, there are ways to prepare the hair to be more accepting to henna, Carryl says. Recipes can be tailored to meet a particular hair type and need. If your hair is dry, adding shea butter can be a great addition. If your focus is on color and gray coverage, adding aloe vera can add moisture without diluting coverage.

Henna will vary in color depending upon where it comes from. For example, in Morocco, the henna has a faster dye release with a more copper tone. Henna coming from India tends to be more burgundy or auburn in tone. Some hennas are creamier, while others have a stringier texture. She urges people to use body-art quality henna powder because it has the highest dye content and will give the best results.

One aspect of henna to be aware of: Using a traditional colorant after using henna can be problematic. Henna coats the hair shaft and can prevent the chemicals in a traditional colorant from penetrating the hair shaft and processing properly.

Additionally, "henna is a permanent hair color so it doesn't wash out or go away," Carryl cautions. "It will stay in the hair until it grows out. The benefits of henna—the shine and protection of each strand—will fade due to washing, product use, and the elements."

FANTASY COLOR

> "I color my hair every 3-4 months, I just let the roots grow out until I'm ready to change the color again. I usually decide my next color based on the current season, the up and coming season or sometimes my mood. LOL."
>
> —RHEA CARTER, FASHION BLOGGER

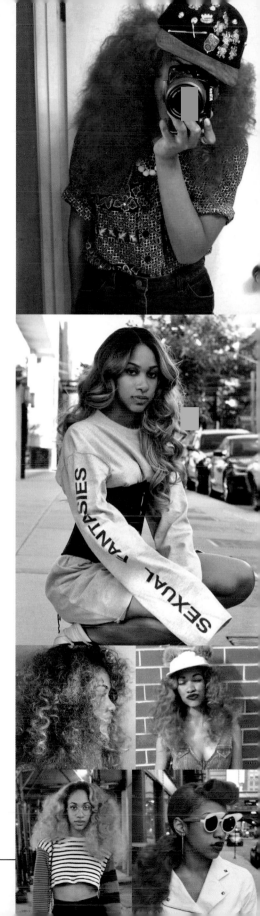

If you look at social media, you'll see curly influencers rocking a rainbow of colors these days. If you're feeling the urge to try a vibrant color like purple, blue, or red, there are some things you should consider before you jump in.

If you want to get pastel or vibrant locks, then you will most likely need to lighten your hair before coloring in order for the dye to show up. Unless you already have very light, blonde hair, the color simply will not show up on your strands, which will make bleaching or double-processing a necessary step in the process. Unfortunately, lightening and coloring can cause breakage, higher porosity, and more dryness.

There are many color options on the market when it comes to blues, purples, and pinks, but you'll find that most of them are temporary. Depending on how vibrant you want your color to be, you can mix a small amount—start with just one drop—of a purple dye with 2 cups of conditioner to create a lavender tint. If you want the color to be darker or more vibrant, you can add more color to your mixture until it resembles your desired color. You can also add small amounts of blue or pink to alter the resulting color.

COVERING GRAY

"How come there are still little bits of gray that still show up even after a fresh dye? Is it like I heard and the gray hairs won't take color, or did the colorist not leave it on enough or something like that?"

Gray hair can be frustrating, no matter what your hair texture. But for curlies it has its own special challenges. Because of the hair's porosity, gray hair can be very stubborn, McLemore says.

Why does your hair go gray? Your body produces a protein called melanin, which allows your hair to grow in (at the root) through melanin-filled cells. At some point (usually in your early thirties, though it can happen much sooner), your body stops producing this protein, resulting in a lack of melanocytes. Your melanocytes share melanin with keratinocytes, which produce keratin. When the keratinocytes die off, they still hold onto the melanin, which means they're hanging on to your hair color. As a result, new hair that grows in has no pigment and presents itself as gray or white.

A single-process permanent color can be used successfully to cover gray. Gray stands out more dramatically in black and brown tones, but it's also easier to cover because darker dyes are absorbed best by gray hair. For blondes and redheads, grays aren't as visible and can actually look like subtle highlights.

To help blend gray hair, rather than completely cover it, you can strategically place both highlights and lowlights. "This approach can help them grow out their gray more forgivingly versus having to go cold turkey," Harbinger says. "It allows them to embrace their gray hair in baby steps. I call it a transition highlight or lowlight."

There also are a number of temporary options available to cover gray roots. They are available in powder and aerosol options.

So what do you do with the "twangers"— those wiry gray hairs that don't match the natural texture of your curls or coils? One Curltalker described her gray hairs as "wiry little devils that are like an unkempt horse mane/tail." A little gel on the tip of your fingers can tame these wayward grays.

COLORING TIPS FOR DO-IT-YOURSELFERS

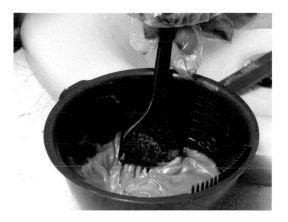

If you're about to color your hair at home, take a moment and read through these tips to help you get the best possible results.

Know Your Hair

Know how to analyze color and texture. Examine the texture, porosity, condition, and color possibilities before you apply the color.

Get It In Shape

Make sure your hair is trimmed and in good condition. Deep condition before coloring to ensure your hair has proper moisture, and do it at least 24 hours before you color to ensure that the cuticle isn't coated. If the cuticle is coated, color won't penetrate the cortex.

Seek Inspiration

Look at Pinterest, Instagram, YouTube, and your favorite hair sites and blogs to see all the color options out there. Never has there been a time when curly girls have been more creative when it comes to color.

Read Instructions—Carefully!

If you're coloring at home, take your time to make sure you fully comprehend the manufacturer's directions. "Make sure you understand the process before you dive right in," says Stephanie McLemore, Dark & Lovely lead style squad member.

Most boxes will tell you how a particular shade will look with your own hair color, although there might be variations depending upon the condition of your hair. If you have questions, most brands include a phone number you can call to talk to someone who can assist you.

Proper Application Is Key

Although this may vary depending upon your hair, you should apply the color first to the middle of your hair, then to the new growth at your scalp, and finally to your ends.

"All three areas may take color differently," McLemore says.

Beware of Layering

Over time, applying the same color over hair that's already colored can result in the midlength and ends looking dark, dull, and muddy. It's important to focus on the regrowth, and to adjust the color you apply to take into account the color that's already on your hair.

Color During the Day

Professional hair expert Scott Cornwall, creator of the Scott Cornwall Colour Restore line, says artificial lights can mute and alter depths and tones and prevent you from thoroughly checking development. You will only see the hair's true color result in natural light.

Use a Tint Bowl

Always use a tint bowl and brush and never apply a color directly from the applicator bottle, Cornwall says. Using a color brush will give you precision and ensure the hair is covered accurately. If you simply pour the color directly from the applicator bottle onto the head, you can cause a patchy or uneven result.

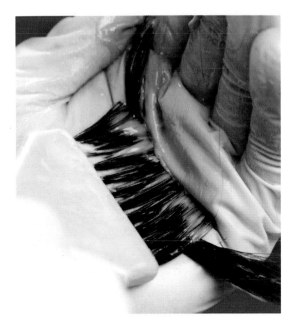

Cool It

Always rinse and shampoo hair with cool water. This helps close the cuticle and prevents color fading.

Say Goodbye to Sulfates

As we've outlined in other chapters, sulfates can be drying to your hair. While there's not a lot of scientific evidence showing that sulfates strip hair color, there's plenty of anecdotal evidence that they can cause color to fade.

Buy Enough Product

Make sure you have enough product for your hair. A head of curls or coils can require more color than usual, so you may need more than one box. This is especially true if your hair is thick and porous.

Buy the Right Product

Not all at-home hair color is for every service. Formulas designed to cover gray are formulated differently than other types of color, McLemore says. If you're unsure, you should go to a professional stylist.

Drastic Change? Go to a Salon

You'll be able to look at color swatches and see what will look best with your skin tone. Some colors may require the use of a bleach or lightener, which is best left to a professional who has experience with these kinds of color processes and can assess exactly how to achieve a certain look. Sometimes the color you want may not be the right shade for you, and a trained colorist can help you find the look that will be most flattering.

Some women decide to forgo coloring their gray hair altogether, either from the first time a gray strand pops up, or after some period of coloring.

For the latter group, the decision to go gray is often because they are fed up with the demarcation line of their gray hair and the colored hair, and the time, effort, and money required to cover it.

Going gray shouldn't be viewed as throwing in the towel. For many women, silver curls are a flattering option. In fact, one stylist we work with calls her gray clients her "silver sirens."

Trae Bodge, a smart shopper/lifestyle writer, started going gray in her twenties. Initially, she would pluck the grays out. But they would always come back in. "I noticed gray hair started coming in on the sides and it looked kind of cool. It was kind of interesting to see what happens."

Bodge says attitudes have changed significantly over the past 25 years. "So many people are embracing it now," she asserts.

But not everyone.

As more gray came in, she got interesting responses. Some women were very disapproving. She says stylists have told her it was "aging" and have offered to "fix it."

A year ago, she had a conversation with a celebrity hairstylist who was bothered by her gray hair. "We were having a lovely lunch and out of nowhere, he was like, 'What's the deal with your hair?' I said, 'I think it's cool.'"

She has no desire to cover it. "It's been one of the aspects of aging that I've enjoyed. Now that I have so much of it, I don't think I could see myself any other way."

Bodge says going gray isn't for everyone. "Gray is a tricky color (or absence of color) and it doesn't suit everyone," she says.

Her advice is to let it grow in a bit and see how it looks instead of fighting it right off the bat.

"It may grow in in a great pattern that is super flattering or it may not," she says.

If you're not crazy about where the streaks are coming in, go to an experienced colorist to get suggestions about how to work with it. To enhance her gray, she adds darker lowlights every 12 weeks.

"Women need to change how they think of gray," Bodge says. "Look around! There are so many people out there who are totally rocking their gray, and you can too!"

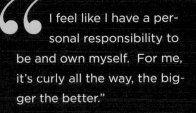

" I feel like I have a personal responsibility to be and own myself. For me, it's curly all the way, the bigger the better."

—Trae Bodge, smart shopping/ lifestyle expert and founder of TraeBodge.com

Texture: 3b/3c, low porosity, fine, thick

Regimen: I wash my hair once every four days. I use DPHUE Apple Cider Vinegar Hair Rinse and use Bumble and Bumble Curl Custom Conditioner at the ends, I towel dry, and I put in Naturelle Luxe Majestic Oil Ultra Hydrating Styling Cream and CVS Nuance Selma Hayak Blue Agave Curl Cream. I combine those, let my hair get close to dry, and blow-dry it to loosen up the curls. I don't diffuse.

"Depending on how strenuous your workouts may be, I suggest braids or twists. If your workouts are light, don't be afraid to rock your natural hair. Tie your edges up with a scarf so you can look fresh."

—Asia Brazil, bikini bodybuilder

Texture: 3c/4b, high porosity, coarse, thick

Regimen: I use Taliah Waajid Clean-n-Curly Hydrating Shampoo, Kenra Curl Styling Conditioner, and Taliah Waajid The Great Detangler. For edge control, I'll add Crème of Nature with Argan Oil Perfect Edges and Taliah Waajid Curly Curl Cream, and DevaCurl Mist-er Right.

Chapter 9

CURL CHALLENGES AND THEIR SOLUTIONS

Curls and coils have a personality of their own. Your hair may be dry and break easily. It may be highly sensitive to the weather, shrinking and frizzing at the slightest rise in humidity. And it can easily tangle, ending up in tiny knots.

"Curly hair can be extremely challenging due to its inconsistent texture," says celebrity curl expert Christo of Christo Fifth Avenue. "One head of curly hair can have 4 to 8 different types of curl patterns."

Knowledge is power when it comes to working with your texture. Understanding that there are solutions to your challenges can empower you to embrace your curls, coils, and waves.

FRIZZ: THE CURLY GIRL'S DREADED 5-LETTER WORD

A stylist once explained that 10 hairs together make a curl and 10 hairs apart equal frizz. While this is a great analogy, it's not necessarily as simple as that.

For many curly and wavy girls, frizz can be their most dreaded issue—a constant source of frustration and one of the biggest obstacles to loving your curls. Frizz can rob your curls of shine and shape and, worst of all, make your hair look dry, damaged, and unhealthy even if it's not.

> **"I love curly hair and I would love for mine to be beautiful, strong, and healthy. But on the contrary, I always have crown frizz, poufy semi-defined curls, and it gradually puffs up throughout the day."**
>
> — 2B CURLTALKER

What exactly is frizz and why is it so commonplace among curlyheads? To understand frizz, let's first consider what your curls look like when they are "frizz-free." Words like "defined" and "shiny" come to mind. These traits describe your curls when the curl pattern is clumped together rather than separated into individual strands all going in a different direction.

"Frizz is excessive misalignment of the hair," says Erica Douglas, a cosmetic chemist who goes by the name "Sister Scientist."

What causes your curls to separate? Porosity plays a big role. The cuticle is made up of overlapping protein scales that resemble the bark of a tree or shingles on the roof of a house. The way these scales lift and close controls how much water goes into and out of your hair and determines your hair's moisture balance. In straight hair, the cuticle tends to lay smooth and flat. If your hair is highly porous, the scales are naturally raised.

Unfortunately, this lifted state of your cuticle predisposes your hair to puffiness for two reasons. First, it allows internal moisture to escape (another reason why curly hair tends to be dry), and second, it allows moisture from the environment to pass through your hair. This is why a rainy or humid day can spell disaster for curls.

"Frizz is often triggered by the hair being exposed to humidity or moisture, which lifts the cuticle," Douglas says. "Hydrogen bonds in the hair become attracted to the hydrogen bonds in water molecules in the air. This moisture swells the strands, and poof—hello, frizz."

Of course, there are many other factors besides the weather that impact frizz, including your texture type. The curlier your hair texture, the more naturally open your cuticle is and the more prone it is to frizz, notes Jonathan Torch.

There's also the health of your curls to consider. Anything that opens the cuticle contributes to frizz. Chemical processes like hair color and relaxers permanently damage the cuticle layer and often leave hair in a frayed and frizzy state. Heat styling with flat irons or curling irons also damages the cuticle layer. Even seemingly innocent habits—such as using a towel or brushing your hair—are no-nos for curlies because heat and friction can rough up your cuticle and contribute to frizz.

Product application can significantly affect frizz. If the product is not applied evenly, it can interfere with the clumping that creates curl definition. That's why the technique you use to apply your styling product can be a huge factor in whether your curls turn to frizz.

The right haircut is also essential for keeping frizz under control. It should encourage curl formation. Thinning shears and razors—which are used by some stylists to reduce bulk—can be a disaster in the wrong hands, resulting in even more bulk and frizz.

You can take steps to prevent frizz from sabotaging your style, and use techniques that fight frizz throughout the day. Unfortunately, there's no permanent solution to frizz, especially if you live in a humid environment or have tighter coils. But the right tricks can arm you with the power to control it.

FRIZZ-FIGHTING SOLUTIONS

Don't Over Cleanse

Cleansing our hair every day is actually bad for our curls, coils, and waves. If you are using shampoo (even a sulfate-free shampoo) every day, you are heading toward drying your hair out. Our hair needs those natural oils, which help prevent frizz and breakage.

Keep Your Hair Hydrated

When your curls are thirsty, they seek out moisture from the atmosphere, so it's important to keep your hair regularly nourished with conditioners, deep treatments, and leave-in conditioners that are appropriate for your texture type. Comb your conditioner through your hair with a wide-tooth comb. Similarly, you need to avoid over-cleansing and using shampoo formulas that rob your hair of natural oils and leave the cuticle vulnerable to frizz.

"Hair can be frizzy because it is reaching out into the atmosphere for moisture," says Robin Sjoblom. "Always apply some type of 'filler'—a foam, milk, or cream that fills the hair with moisture so the curls remain frizz-free—to the curl before adding a gel."

Use Frizz-Fighting Products

Use an anti-humectant styling product to prevent moisture in the air from entering the hair shaft and causing strands to expand and lose definition. Look for products with ingredients such as lanolin, beeswax, and water-soluble silicones. Depending upon your hair and its porosity, it may take a combination of two or more products for the best frizz protection. Your texture type—and lots of trial and error—will determine which is the best frizz-fighting cocktail to use.

Product Application Is Key

For best frizz-fighting results, make sure your hair is soaking wet when you apply your styling product. As it starts to dry, it's harder to encourage the clumping that creates defined curls. You can also end up looking frizzy if you rush through your application or miss some spots. You need to evenly coat your curls to get maximum definition. To do this, divide your hair into sections, especially if you have a lot of hair. Then use your fingers to pull the product from root to end, ensuring that every strand is lightly coated.

To distribute product evenly, Vazquez has found that putting plastic wrap or gloves on her hands when applying product also helps eliminate frizz.

"Sometimes we don't know how to control the amount of pressure we are applying to curly hair," Vazquez explains. "This provides a smoother application on the hair and lessens the amount of frizz while it's drying."

Some CurlTalk community members use the "Praying Hands" Method, which involves cocktailing your styling product into your palms and running your hands—one on each side, matched as in prayer—over your lengths of hair, section by section.

Air-Dry Whenever Possible

Blasting your curls with hot air from a blow-dryer is a great way to make your curls poof up like a frizz ball, not to mention cause heat damage to your cuticle. Ideally, you want to allow your curls to dry naturally. If that's not an option, a diffuser attachment or hood dryer is a good alternative. It will circulate air without disturbing your curl pattern or disrupting your cuticle.

Avoid "Regular" Fabrics

Did know that using a cotton bath towel or pillowcase can make your curls extra puffy? It may sound like a tiny detail, but it can make a big difference! These fabrics have tiny nubs that will fluff up your cuticle layer, setting you up for a frizzy day. Minimize post-shower friction by blotting wet curls with a microfiber towel or a T-shirt and wrap your curls in a silk scarf or sleep on a satin pillowcase to avoid unnecessary roughness at nighttime.

Pack a Frizz Emergency Kit

Frizz can be sneaky. No matter how well you condition or prep your curls, there's always that random situation when you find yourself unexpectedly puffy. Experienced curlies are always prepared with a travel-size version of a favorite smoothing product, and/or a portable styling tool to calm down frizzies. And it's always good to have a Plan B in case the elements are too much: a ponytail holder, a headband, a turban.

Don't Touch!

Don't touch your hair even though it's tempting! The more you play with and tousle your hair during the day, the more frizz you're going to get. You can perform a midday touch up by moistening broken curls and wrapping them around your finger to reshape them.

Accept it!

Curl expert Shai Amiel— the "Curl Doctor"—explains to his clients that frizz is a natural part of curly hair, and is not a bad thing. "With proper hair care the frizz can be minimized and we get the 'happy frizz' that actually makes it look cool and textured,' says the owner of Capella Salon in Los Angeles.

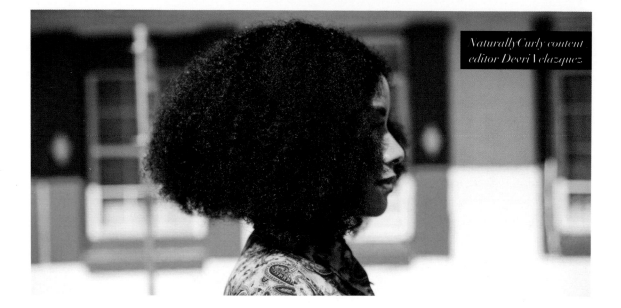

NaturallyCurly content editor Devri Velazquez

THE BEAUTY OF FRIZZ

We've seen all of the ads promising: "How to Fight the Frizz" or "Defrizz Your Hair Fast." For many women with tight coils, the topic of frizz can be frustrating and insulting. Especially since the word is almost always used in a negative way. For many type 4 coily women, frizz isn't something to be dreaded.

Frizz is beautiful, flossy, puffy, voluminous, and ethereal. Frizz *is* the style. By creating the perception that all women want defined curls, the beauty industry has done a huge disservice to all the women for whom frizz is the glorious look of their hair in its natural state.

"Frizz is the reason why textured hair has so much volume," says texture expert Diane Da Costa, author of *Textured Tresses: The Ultimate Guide to Maintaining and Styling Natural Hair*. "Frizz is the key to enhancing the Big Afro."

It may take time for the word "frizz" to lose its negative connotation, but it's already happening, thanks in part to vocal and empowered naturalistas who are expanding the standard of beauty.

"I call myself unapologetically frizzy because I love the aspect of frizz and curls living together," says stylist Isabella Vazquez. "It's beautiful. It's eye candy. It is a gorgeous texture."

SHRINKAGE

> "Can anyone give me some advice on shaping hair with TONS of shrinkage? My hair is almost belly-button length when it's stretched out but shoulder length when it's completely dry."
>
> —4A CURLTALKER

Shrinkage is a fact of life for women with curls and coils, and the tighter the curl, the more shrinkage you are likely to experience. Some only have 20–30 percent shrinkage while others may see their hair shrink by as much as 75 percent! Our hair expands when wet and shrinks while drying.

When you pull a curl down just to see it snap back up, it can be frustrating for those wanting length. There are several ways you can achieve a stretched look with your curls, including styling methods that stretch the hair to reduce shrinkage. They include braid-out, banding, bunning, roller sets, and twists.

DRYNESS

> "Suddenly my hair has become really dried out! Especially the surface layer of my hair. I was so surprised because it's been in great shape so far this winter."
>
> –3A CURLTALKER

By its nature, textured hair has a hard time retaining moisture throughout the entire length of the strand when compared to straight hair. The ends become especially dry and brittle, and because of this, many curlies must regularly trim their hair to get rid of those dry ends.

But several factors may make our hair drier than it should be. One of those is improper product use, says celebrity texture guru Pekela Riley. She cites the improper use of oils as a key factor. While many use oils to add moisture, the molecules in most oils are too large to pass through the cuticle of the hair. Instead the oil may actually be creating a barrier that prevents the hair from absorbing moisture. You want to make sure you are using oil after the hair has been properly moisturized with a water-based product.

"Oil can seal moisture, but (in most cases) it's not moisture," Riley says. "You should be moisturizing with creams and water-based products, and then sealing with oil."

Overuse of proteins can also cause dryness for some women. That is because the hair is predominantly made of protein, which provides it with strength and structure. When you apply too much protein, the hair can harden, making it feel dry and, in some cases, leading to breakage. If you're experiencing dryness, look at the ingredients in your hair products to see if they contain a hydrolyzed protein. If so, you may want to limit your use of products that contain that ingredient.

Although some types of alcohols—like fatty alcohols—moisturize the hair, others can be very drying, including SD alcohol 40, ethanol alcohol, propyl alcohol, SD alcohol, propanol alcohol, and isopropyl alcohol.

Are you flat ironing or regularly blowing out your hair? If you are and you're not using a heat protectant, that could be drying out your hair. Each shaft of hair has 7 to 12 layers of cuticle scales. Their job is to protect the inside of the shaft, known as the cortex. Excessive use of heat will create cracks and damage the cuticle as well as blistering and fracturing the hair.

Sulfates, which are in many traditional shampoos, can dry out the hair and should be used sparingly. Sulfates you should avoid include sodium lauryl sulfate, sodium laureth sulfate, and ammonium laurel sulfate.

Dryness can vary by the season. In the winter, when humidity is low and heaters are cranked up inside, hair can become dehydrated. In the summer, the combination of intense sun, salt water in the ocean, and chlorine can be especially drying.

Make sure you're deep conditioning regularly—how often depends on the condition of your hair. For best results, you need some heat to help open the cuticle of the hair so the conditioner soaks in. You may need to experiment with various deep conditioners that contain different ingredients to find the one that works best for your hair.

BREAKAGE

> **"I have noticed a considerable amount of breakage and extreme dryness. Do you have any suggestions on preventing hair breakage and dryness?"**
>
> —3C CURLTALKER

Many women are distressed by the amount of hair they shed in the shower daily. But, are you losing your hair or are you actually experiencing hair breakage?

When your hair naturally falls from the root, you are experiencing hair loss. Some amount of hair loss is normal and to be expected. In fact, while you may not be aware of it, you're likely losing up to 100 strands a day.

Breakage is most noticeable when brushing or combing your hair, removing a hair band, or in the shower. Breakage and dryness can go hand in hand. The drier the hair, the more prone it is to breakage. But there are other factors as well that can cause breakage.

Managing it roughly, especially when it's wet, is a leading cause of breakage, says Riley. "When it's wet, it's fragile; you have a temporary fault line."

To prevent this, take extra care in the detangling process. Use a wide-tooth comb, and determine the method that works best for you. For some this will involve coating your strands with a high-slippage conditioner and combing in the shower, while for others this may be finger detangling afterward.

Chemical services like bleaching and relaxers as well as daily heat styling also can damage the hair, leading to breakage. Even heat-free styles that involve a lot of tension can result in breakage. Whether you're wearing a bun, braids, cornrows, or faux locs, make sure to use the least amount of tension possible. Too often, people make their styles tight in the belief it will make their style last longer.

"I want to debunk the myth that tighter means longer," Riley says. "You don't gain additional days, and you risk follicle damage and breakage."

Many women have hair that's predestined to break, Riley says. They aren't getting enough of the nutrients they need to grow healthy, strong hair. Make sure you're eating a balanced diet.

SINGLE-STRAND KNOTS (SSK)

> "My hair is driving me crazy. Everywhere I look I see fairy knots or split ends, and I assume breakage because my hair is a million different lengths (which makes it tremendously frustrating to give myself dusting trims)."
>
> —3C CURLTALKER

Single strand knots (also known as SSKs), also known as fairy knots, can be the bane of a curly girl's existence. Fairy knots are actual strands of hair that knot within themselves and often add other adjoining hairs into the mix, creating even bigger knots. They tend to create tiny balls at the ends of our hair that seem to spring up overnight. Most people see them as an unavoidable fact of life, while others seek out ways to prevent them.

You can rub some conditioner between your thumb and index finger on the fairy knot to release some if not all of the hairs in the knot. Removing them with your fingers is better than trying with a comb or brush, which could just remove the knot along with other perfectly healthy hairs in the process.

HAIR VITAMINS: FEEDING THE HAIR FROM WITHIN

A nutritious, balanced diet is one of the biggest factors that impacts the health and growth rate of your hair. But not everyone has the time nor the discipline to chow down 10 carrots every day in order to fill up on vitamin A. That's why many women with curls and coils are turning to hair vitamins, and why it's become one of the hottest product categories.

Experts agree that hair vitamins can promote hair health, including strengthening hair and reducing breakage, by addressing vitamin deficiencies. A hair vitamin contains specific vitamins that are only absorbed by the cells in our hair follicles and cuticles (with some others that are good for our overall health as well). All hair types can only benefit from getting the extra nutrients—and your outcome is not only thicker, stronger hair, but also an improved complexion, nail growth, and nail strength with less chipping.

Hair vitamins include some or all of the the following: Vitamin A, Biotin, Niacin, Vitamin B5 (Pantothenic Acid), Folic Acid, Vitamin C, and Vitamin E.

PYRAMID HEAD/ TRIANGLE HEAD

> **"I recently got my hair cut (a curly bob style) and now I have flat-top, pyramid looking hair. I don't know what to do."**
>
> —CURLTALKER

Pyramid head is one the most common complaints among curlies. The triangular shape is caused by hair that's flat on the top but bulky at the ends. Cutting and styling solutions can eliminate this issue.

Ouidad says pyramid head is common when a stylist doesn't understand how to cut curly hair. It usually results when the hair is cut bluntly with no angles or layers. "They're doing a straight haircut on a curly girl thinking they are going to blow it out. This is a stylist who truly doesn't understand a curl pattern," she says.

A cut that creates strategic layering and sculpting of the curls will give you the volume you want on the surface of the hair and more length on the bottom.

When styling the hair, use DevaClips at the roots to create lift at the crown to keep the hair from weighing itself down, says Shari Harbinger, cofounder of DevaCurl Academy.

To clip your roots, take two fingers and lift one family of curls near the base of the scalp and place the clip as close to—or on—the scalp horizontally, Harbinger says. Use 6–10 clips. Try not to touch the damp hair during the drying process as touching often results in frizz.

CHEMO CURLS

> **"I am a year after my last chemo treatment for breast cancer. My hair was very fine and straight before, and never grew past my shoulders. Now I have this still very short but curly and thick hair. I have no idea what to do. I look like an 80-year-old woman with a new perm. Please help me."**
>
> —CURLTALKER

Cancer can be a terrifying, life-changing diagnosis. The hair loss caused by chemotherapy makes the cancer even more real, and can deal an emotional blow.

"I work with many cancer patients, and have seen firsthand how it affects them," says integrative medicine practitioner Dr. Shimeca Videau. "Hair is an essential part of most women's lives and when that is compromised, it can affect them deeply."

The hair loss occurs over a period of days or weeks and may include hair loss on the entire body, including eyebrows and eyelashes. Regrowth, which usually occurs six to eight weeks after treatment ends, can pose its own challenges. In many cases, the hair that grows back may be dramatically different in texture and color than the hair that was lost—at least in the short term.

"Chemo curls" are a common phenomenon among cancer patients who've undergone chemotherapy. Some of our readers first discovered NaturallyCurly in their quest to learn what to do with their new head of curls after a lifetime of having straight or wavy hair.

Chemo curls can be new and exciting if you've always wanted curly hair. They can also be a big pain if you've never had curls, never wanted curls, and are fighting the urge to press your hair between the plates of a flat iron.

What causes chemo curls? When chemotherapy enters the body, it attacks and kills the fast-growing cancer cells. But chemotherapy drugs also attack other fast-growing cells, including the ones responsible for hair growth. (Different chemotherapy drugs have different hair-loss effects.) In the short term,

the chemo can damage the cells that determine hair texture. Once chemotherapy completely exits the body, cell production usually reverts back to what it was pre-chemo.

It is important to treat the new hair with a great deal of TLC, says curl pioneer and cancer survivor Ouidad.

Ouidad recommends using a deep conditioner every two weeks. It is also important to get a trim every 10 to 12 weeks to keep the new growth looking its best. As for color, she says, it's better to wait a while. She recommends that women wait at least six months to color their hair after chemo treatments to allow the hair roots to strengthen.

Some cancer survivors learn to embrace their chemo curls, and actually miss them a little when their hair reverts back to its pre-chemo texture.

> **"I'm loving my chemo curls, but I'll go with the flow. When it's straight again, I'll love that, too!"**
>
> —AN ANONYMOUS BREAST CANCER SURVIVOR

WORKING OUT

Exercise indisputably does wonders for our bodies and minds. Unfortunately, sweating and swimming can pose a challenge to our curls and coils. In some cases, textured hair actually prevents women from committing to a regular workout routine. It shouldn't, especially with the tremendous health benefits provided by exercise.

Many of us curlies exercise on a regular basis, and we've found ways to make it work.

"You are at your most beautiful when you're fully alive, energetic, and strong," says peloton instructor, personal trainer, and author Nicole Meline. "Perfect hair is a lousy trade. I think sweat is the fountain of youth. Sweat hard once a day. There are so many ways of rocking your hair during and after a workout. So blaze!"

Meline acknowledges that there might be more curl-friendly exercises than running, swimming, or cycling, but the trade-off isn't worth it for her. "I do all the 'wrong' workouts for curls—spinning, road biking (helmet hair!), swimming (caps, chlorine!), hot yoga—with a vengeance. Work out like crazy and let your hair be crazier."

Here are some tips for working out:

Cleansing Isn't Necessary

Even after the sweatiest workout, you don't necessarily have to shampoo your hair. A perfect alternative to washing is just rinsing, conditioning, and leaving it alone. There are also great products on the market that can freshen it up, such as curl refreshers and dry shampoos.

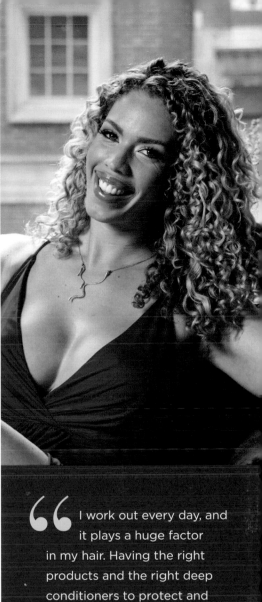

" I work out every day, and it plays a huge factor in my hair. Having the right products and the right deep conditioners to protect and condition is really important."

—Layla Luciano, fitness professional/model

Texture: 3b, high porosity, coarse, thick

Regimen: I use Curlisto Structura Lotion, Control Gel II, Curlisto Protein Boost, and Cantu Coconut Curling Cream.

> "I've embraced my curls. I let them get big and huge and crazy. It informs my look and style. I'll always have this big, crazy curly hair."

—Nicole Meline, athlete, trainer, and writer

Texture: 3b/3c, high porosity, fine, thick

Regimen: I use Ouidad Moisture Lock Leave-in Conditioner, Ouidad Deep Treatment Curl Restoration Masque, and a cocktail of Ouidad Climate Control Heat & Humidity Gel and Tigi Curls Rock Curlesque Curls Rock Curl Amplifier.

Find Fitness-Friendly Hair Styles

Some women opt for braids or twists that enable them to go seamlessly between workout and work. Buns are also a good option—providing benefits similar to pineappling. (See styling techniques.)

Protect It!

If you swim regularly, you will want to protect your hair from the drying effects of chlorine. Before going in the pool, slather your hair (wet or dry) with a rich conditioner. Curly hair is porous, so the conditioner fills those holes before the chlorine can seep in. Next, slip on a bathing cap.

After a swim, whether it's in the pool or the ocean, rinse your hair immediately with a sulfate-free cleanser or conditioner to remove any drying chlorine or salt water.

Loosen Up; No Tight Ponytail

To keep your curl pattern intact, you can twist your hair loosely and keep it in place with a scrunchie or a hair tie that won't leave a dent or stretch out limp curls.

Accessorize

A good way to absorb sweat and keep your hair off your face is to use a thick cotton headband, scarf, or turban. "I think of them as functional tiaras," Meline says.

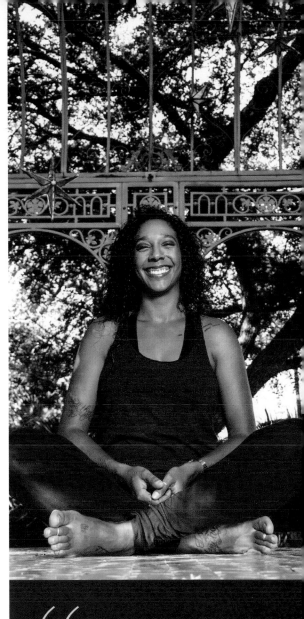

" I wear it up a lot with hair ties."
—**Keeley Crowfoot, psychologist, yogi**

Texture: 3b/3c, high porosity, coarse, thick

Regimen: I use baking soda as a shampoo and coconut oil as a conditioner. I have a jar in my shower.

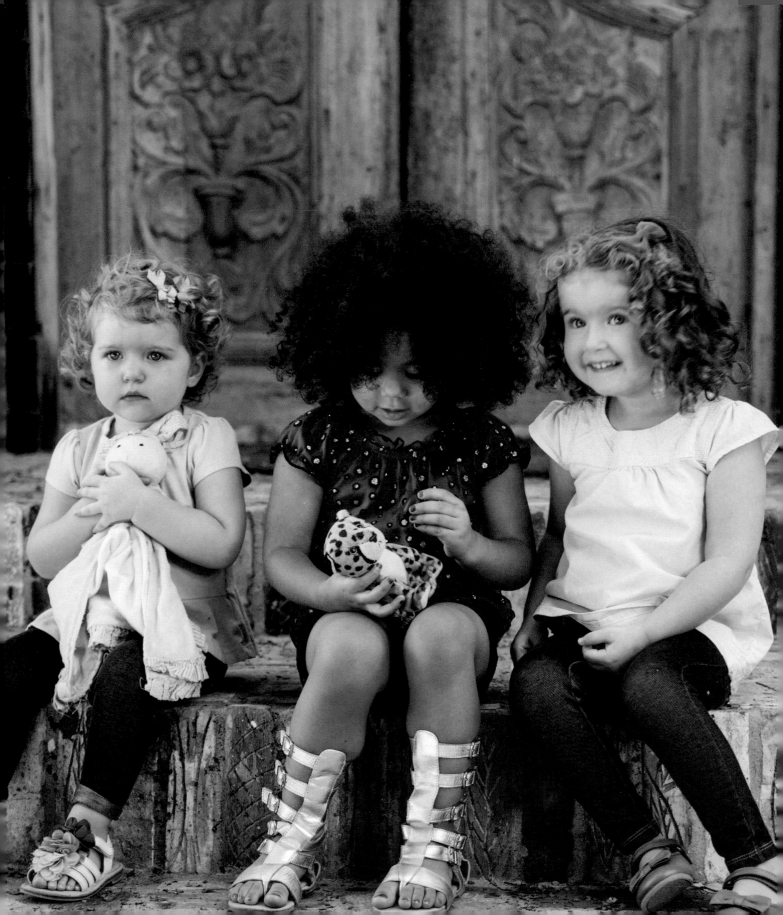

Chapter 10

CURLY KIDS —

WHERE IT ALL STARTS

Amanda Crawford will never forget the sight of her then 8-year-old daughter Deborah-Ann coming off the school bus in tears. The second-grader had been viciously teased about her coily hair.

"They told her she had horse hair," Crawford said. "When your kid struggles with something that's such a part of who she is, it's incredibly painful."

Crawford said her daughter—who is biracial—was already unhappy about her hair, which didn't look like either her mother's looser curls or the straight hair of most of her schoolmates. She usually wore it back in a ponytail, slicked down with gel in an attempt to control and hide it.

Her mom took to the Internet and found NaturallyCurly's Facebook page. She showed her daughter examples of confident women with beautiful natural hairstyles.

Deborah-Ann asked her mother to post a picture of her on the Facebook page. Crawford posted the picture, along with the story about the teasing she got about her hair.

The response was overwhelming—and life changing.

That picture got nearly 33,000 likes, 1,400 shares, and 4,800 comments. People

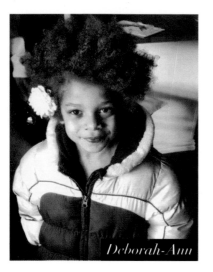
Deborah-Ann

posted words of support, photos of their own daughters and themselves, and stories of their own childhood hair struggles.

"I was crying," Crawford recalls. "I read a lot of the comments to her and she was so tickled. She's turned it around and is so much more confident."

Three years later, Deborah-Ann has become more comfortable with her hair.

"She wants to try more styles now, which is amazing," says Crawford. "She likes to wear it down, have it up in a ponytail, blown out straight, blown out and curled. She recently asked for a frohawk."

A person's perception about their curls begins early.

"I've been in the kids' salon business for 21 years, and it always surprises me how young the kids are when they start to really have an image of themselves and their hair and the role that it plays," says Cozy Friedman, a curly girl and founder of Cozy's Cuts for Kids in New York and the SoCozy product line for kids.

"Everyone jokes about how you feel on a good hair day," says Friedman, a curly girl herself who fought her hair when she was young. "It's no different for kids, because curly hair is a lot harder to manage. I think it adds one more piece to the puzzle."

Before the Curl Revolution, society created a perception that there was only one standard of beauty, and—with the exception of a few icons like Shirley Temple—it usually didn't include curls and coils. It's no wonder that curly kids have grown up fighting their texture when they've grown up with straight-haired Disney princesses and dolls with silky, straight hair.

And then there's the teasing that many curly kids endure on a regular basis. Children can be cruel, and can bully children who look different from them. Hair can often be a target. Many of us curly adults are still shaped by the names we were called as kids—names like Bozo, Frizzy, and Q-Tip.

Parents can play a huge role in boosting their child's self-esteem about their hair.

Children are like little sponges, picking up on everything they see and hear.

"Never say how difficult or unmanageable your child's hair is, even if you become frustrated with it," says Jessica Pettway, a Los Angeles–based mom and beauty influencer.

Lisa Price, founder of the Carol's Daughter hair line, says she's heard parents say, "I don't know what to do with the mess on her head." "It's horrible," she says. "I've actually heard those words."

"Children internalize that as something is wrong with them. They can think 'I'm not pretty, my hair is a problem, I'm an issue. The stuff on my head is a mess,'" Price says. "I've listened to moms say this and I know they don't really mean it in that way. But you could see their children continue to shrink before your eyes and try to look away."

Instead of being negative, focus on what makes curly hair special. Tell your child how beautiful and unique her hair is, and help her find different ways to style it. "Kind of flip it and make it more positive," Price says.

If you have curls or coils yourself, one of the most effective gifts you can give your child is your ability to embrace your own texture.

"They soak up information as well as your energy," Pettway says. "If a child sees their parent appreciating and embracing their hair, they will do the same. This behavior will become normal to them."

Natalie Austin relaxed her hair until five years ago, when she realized she was serving as a role model for her daughter.

"She was asking for straight hair, and I wanted her to be proud of the hair she has. And here I was relaxing my own hair," Austin says. "I don't want her to feel like she has to change herself to be accepted."

Kendra Austin, now 9, says she likes her hair because she can wear it so many different ways, including twist outs, ponytails, and braided pigtails. "Sometimes I like having curly hair and sometimes I can wear it straight. I feel lucky I can go back and forth."

One of the best things you can do is to teach your curly kid how to do her own hair from an early age—as soon as she can hold a wide-tooth comb. Take the time to experiment with techniques and hairstyles to see what works. If you have curly hair, share some of your favorite techniques.

Curl pioneer Ouidad began teaching her daughter, Sondriel, to live a curly lifestyle when she was just a toddler.

"She was 24 months old with her little curls, and I would read to her while we were conditioning our hair with deep treatments," Ouidad says. "If they can help detangle their

> " I started my natural journey three years ago when my daughter saw me relaxing and put her fingers into the relaxer. It's a struggle with both of us being natural. I focus on her right now. I said I was never going to perm her hair until she was old enough to decide what to do."

**— Alise Wheatfall-McIver,
Mother of Caydence, age 10**

Texture: 3c/4a

own hair and they're having fun, they won't have a fear of detangling."

Some salons invite parents and children to visit the salon together to help them learn about curly hair care at the same time.

Whatever your approach, keep it light and positive, says Christo, Global Artistic Director of New York's Christo Fifth Avenue Salon. "From the day your child is born, embrace her curls," Christo says. "Teach her to love who she is and that curly hair is a gift, not a burden."

STRAIGHT PARENT/ CURLY KID

Many straight-haired moms—and dads—have discovered NaturallyCurly when they have a curly kid. They have no personal experience caring for this texture. From haircuts to styling, the rules are completely different.

"We see it all the time, especially with mixed-race marriages," Friedman says. "You could be a Caucasian woman with blonde, straight hair who has a daughter with a full head of really curly, really textured hair. So the trick here is getting information."

For Melissa Romero, who has straight hair, it's been trial and error when it comes to 3-year-old Mia. She likes to try different styles and products, and has discovered a regimen that works to detangle and define Mia's 3c coily curls.

Despite getting complimented all the time about her hair, "she still says she wants straight hair like Elsa in *Frozen*," Romero says. "I tell her that her hair is much prettier than Elsa's in *Frozen*."

There is plenty of help out there for parents; social media, including NaturallyCurly, is loaded with how-to videos and style images.

They may look at your straight, silky hair and wonder why they can't have hair like you. Surround your child with images of people who have texture like hers. While many of us grew up with Barbie dolls with straight blonde hair, there are a growing number of dolls with curly and coily hair.

An inspiring example of one dad's effort to help his daughter embrace her curls came in the form of a Muppet. Joey Mazzarino—a Sesame Street exec—in 2010 created the brown Muppet when his Ethiopian-born daughter bemoaned her natural, "fluffy" hair, wishing instead for flowing "Barbie" hair.

The Muppet sings, "I love my hair. I don't need a trip to the beauty shop, 'cuz I love what I got on top!"

The video went viral. Bloggers wrote that

it brought them to tears because of the message it sends to young black girls. The YouTube video has been viewed more than 6 million times.

Monique Rodriguez, creator of the Mielle hair care line and mother of two curly daughters, grew up straightening her hair. "I didn't think curly was cute," she says. It wasn't until 2012 that she learned how to work with her natural texture.

She wants to help her daughters appreciate their texture rather than spend their lives fighting it like she did. She is always trying different styles and techniques to show them how versatile and beautiful their natural hair is, whether they wear it straight or curly.

"Words matter," Rodriguez says. "Every time I do my daughter's hair, I over-exaggerate. I really want to emphasize that they look pretty no matter how they wear their hair."

TOP TIPS FOR CURLY KIDS

Let Your Child Help

Stand in front of a mirror and show her how you're helping care for her curls. Kids love to exercise their independence, so why not teach them the tricks of the trade, too?

Conditioners Are Your Friend

Use a daily conditioner every time you cleanse. And then use a leave-in conditioner for thicker hair to help avoid knots and tangled hair. Leave-in conditioners can be a key step in keeping little curls looking their best and may help avoid the possible "poof" effect, too.

Hands Off

Tell your little ones to leave their hands off their hair, and hope they'll actually listen! Let them know that fingers in the hair could lead to more combing sessions and extra bath times, both of which lead to less play time—it's true!

Tangle-Free Styles

You may want to put your child's curls in a loose ponytail, or even braid them at night. If your child is active during the day, and still gets lots of tangles, braids and ponytails can be good for those times as well.

Create a Weekend Regimen

Prepping the hair on the weekends will save you time. Create a weekend regimen that

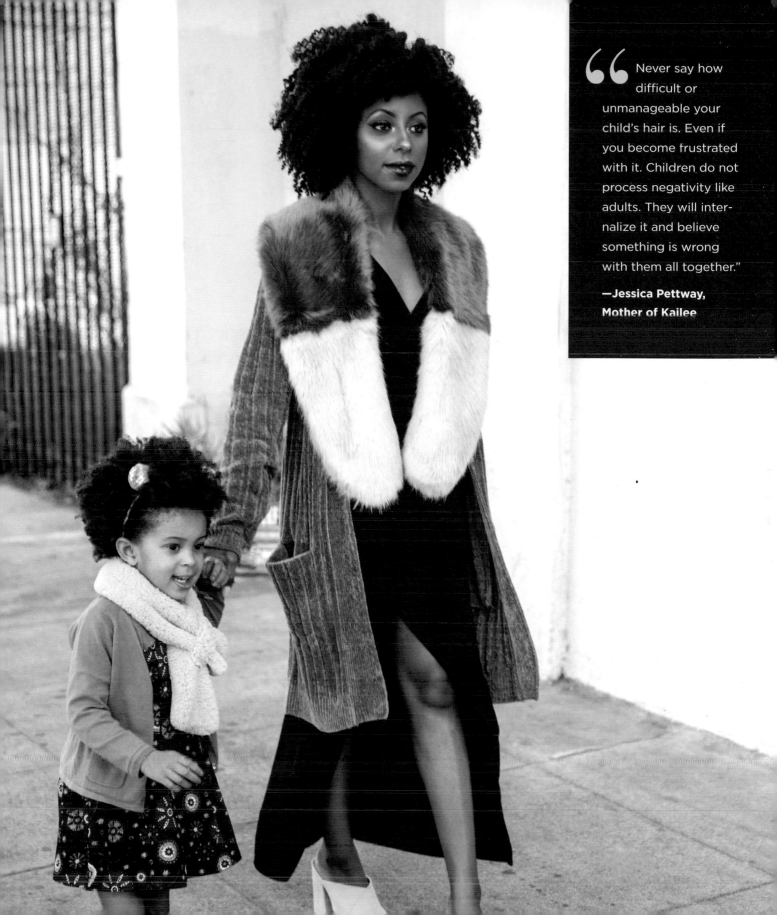

> " Never say how difficult or unmanageable your child's hair is. Even if you become frustrated with it. Children do not process negativity like adults. They will internalize it and believe something is wrong with them all together."
>
> —Jessica Pettway,
> Mother of Kailee

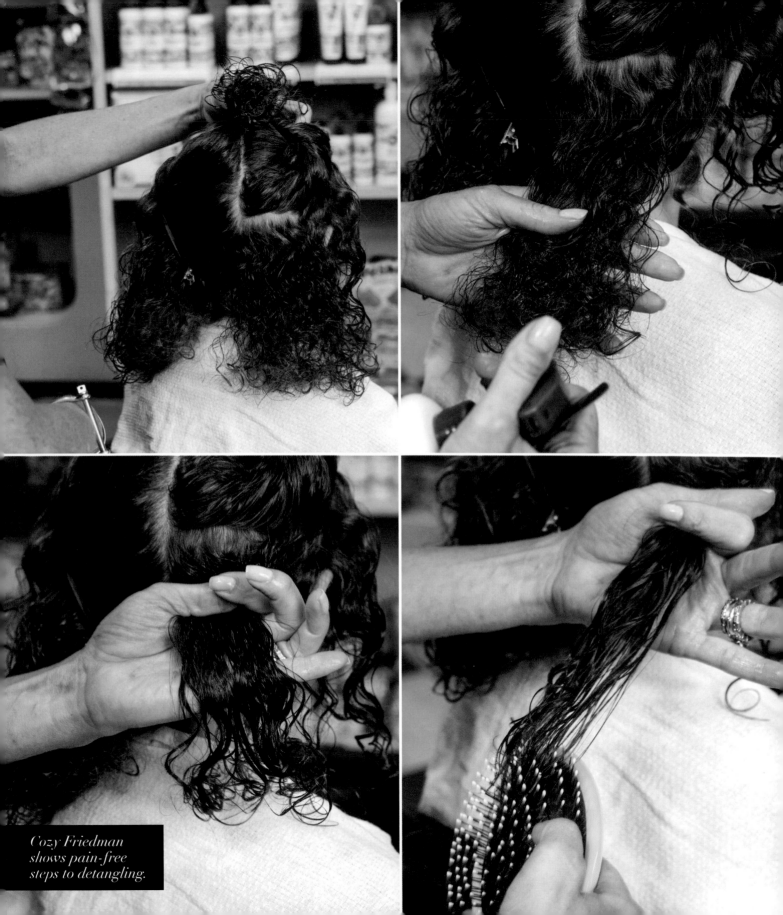

Cozy Friedman shows pain-free steps to detangling.

works for your schedule. Because children are so active, protective styles like twists and braids are great!

DETANGLING TIPS

Detangle in the Tub

The best time to detangle is when the hair is wet.

Try Detangling Products Specifically Created for Kids

There are now several detangling sprays, shampoos, and conditioners—just for kids— that have extra slip to help those tangles unravel. Many have tear-free formulas that will not irritate kids' eyes or skin. Their ingredients list is pumped up with moisturizers to ensure the children's hair is soft, easy to manage, and tangle-free. This is a must-have investment.

Use Conditioners with Tons of Slip

This is also a must as slip allows those tangles to just glide through. Never skip the conditioning step on wash day, as that will help keep the hairs friction-free.

Sleep on a Satin Pillowcase or Wear a Satin Bonnet

Start introducing them to satin. First off, your child will love it, and secondly it will cut down on dryness and breakage. This is also helpful with deterring tangles, so try a satin pillowcase or a satin bonnet for your toddler.

Use Wide-Tooth Combs and Detangling Brushes

These tools make it much easier—and more painless—to remove tangles without yanking or breaking the hair. Many have cute styles and colors that will make your kid want to use them, and that can also help if she or he wants to aid in their hair care.

Don't Procrastinate

Even if it's difficult, do not put off removing those tangles. It will only get worse. If you see she has had a hard day of play and that her hair is beginning to tangle, take a few minutes with a kid's detangling spray, and work the tangles out with a wide-tooth comb or detangling brush.

Q&A WITH COZY

Cozy Friedman, a curly herself, opened her first Cozy's Cuts for Kids in 1994 in New York to create a place dedicated to meeting the hair care needs of kids. She has since developed the SoCozy Professional Hair care line, including the Boing collection for curly kids.

Question: My 6-year-old daughter has 3b curls, and everyone but her thinks they are beautiful. She was very upset last night because she "hates curly hair" and wants "normal straight hair." I have straightened her hair a few times and every time, she loves it—unfortunately straightening is not an option for us every day.

My husband suggested showing her pictures of celebrities with curly hair and reading more stories with curly-haired characters. Any other suggestions to help her see how beautiful her curls are?

Cozy: I felt the same way about my curls when I was little. I wanted straight hair more than anything and was embarrassed by my natural curls. It wasn't until later in life that I embraced my curls, so I think it's amazing that you want to help her at such a young age.

Your husband's idea is excellent—the more she sees her curls represented in books, toys, on TV, in movies, and other images, the more her sense of self and self-love will grow. Also, there are so many gorgeous curly hair styles out there—try looking through Pinterest and YouTube with her for some hair style inspiration and get her involved with styling and accessory decisions. The more excited she is about her hair, the more she'll love it!

Question: I seem to have birthed a curly, and I know not how! My parents, grandparents, husband, and husband's family all have straight hair. I had cute little ringlets until I was about five and my hair all got cut off, then all I got was the odd wavy bit and kink in an otherwise straight mane. Now, my daughter's hair is wretched! She was a baldy baby when she was born and her hair has taken forever to grow. Suddenly, in the last six months, she's grown curls all over her head. Having no family members with curly hair, I neither know how to classify nor how to take care of it. Help me!

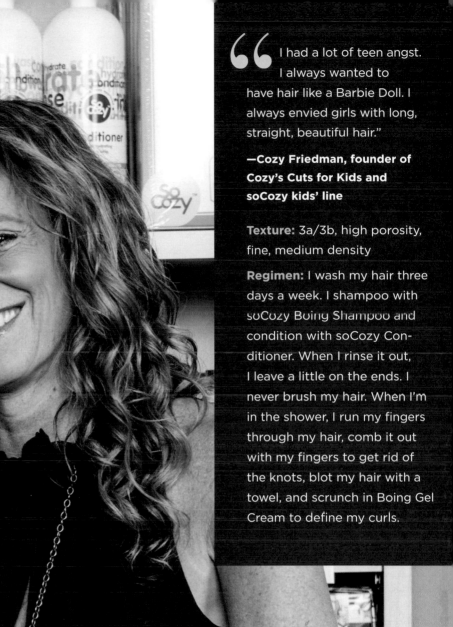

> "I had a lot of teen angst. I always wanted to have hair like a Barbie Doll. I always envied girls with long, straight, beautiful hair."

—Cozy Friedman, founder of Cozy's Cuts for Kids and soCozy kids' line

Texture: 3a/3b, high porosity, fine, medium density

Regimen: I wash my hair three days a week. I shampoo with soCozy Boing Shampoo and condition with soCozy Conditioner. When I rinse it out, I leave a little on the ends. I never brush my hair. When I'm in the shower, I run my fingers through my hair, comb it out with my fingers to get rid of the knots, blot my hair with a towel, and scrunch in Boing Gel Cream to define my curls.

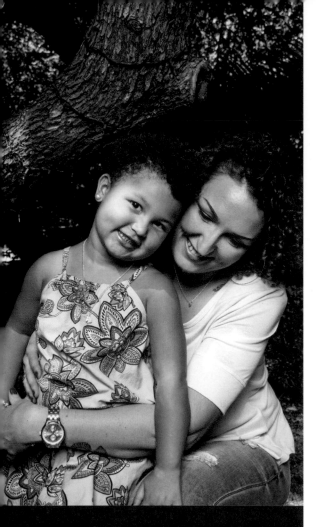

Cozy: Don't worry—a little schooling on curls, and you won't feel like it's a chore anymore. Dry, frizzy curls are usually caused by over-washing hair, which strips hair of its natural oils. Your gut reaction might be to wash her curls often to keep tangles and frizz under control, but you're actually doing the opposite. Try having her go two to three days between washes to allow all of those natural oils to coat and nourish her hair.

Make sure you're using shampoo the right way! Curly hair is a whole different ballgame and different from managing the hair you grew up with. Despite your instinct to use a lot of shampoo, only a dime-size or quarter-size is required.

To keep the spring in her curls, leave-in products work wonders for adding moisture back in, without weighing hair down. While hair is still wet, gently finger-comb her hair from root to tip.

Brushing or untangling dry curls is a no-no. Instead, work in conditioner or use a leave-in. I find that fingers are much easier to comb through curls with, but if you do use a wide-tooth comb, remember to work from tip to root. Now that you've brought your curls to life, make sure you give them some staying power. Work a styling cream, gently scrunch hair, and lift at the root.

Question: My daughters are LOVING the pool! What do you all do to prepare for the pool hair? And what do you do after pool hair? Right now, I don't do any prep. Any suggestions? My daughters have 4a coily and 3b/c curly-coily hair.

Cozy: Using the right products before the pool is just as important as using the products after the pool. My favorite swimming tip is to wet hair with fresh tap water before swimming. Your hair is like a sponge and you want to make sure you're soaking up the good stuff and preventing it from soaking up pool chemicals. It's also a good idea to use a leave-in conditioning spray for added protection before heading outside. After you're done making a splash, make sure you use products formulated to rinse away sun and pool damage.

Question: My 9-year-old is a very restless sleeper. In the morning, her bed is a mess. This has affected her 2a, thick hair. Her hair is usually a mess on the side that she usually sleeps on. It's frizzy and has breakage high up. I tried a satin pillowcase but she usually doesn't stay on her pillow. It is very difficult to make her hair look decent in the morning. Any suggestions?

Cozy: The secret to keeping curls under control while you're sleeping is a simple, loose ponytail or braid. If she's very restless, loop the scrunchie around one extra time just to be sure. This will help minimize the tangles and frizz. In the morning, give her curls a boost by using leave-in conditioner. This will help reshape them and smooth them.

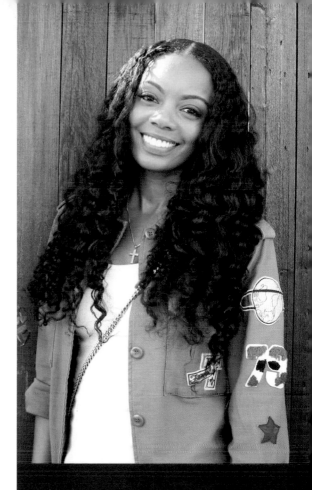

" The best advice I can give my two daughters is to embrace what God gave them. Don't compare their hair texture to someone else's. The best thing you can do is embrace your hair and learn to work with it."

—Monique Rodriguez, founder of Mielle hair care and mother of two daughters

Texture: 3b/3c, medium porosity, fine, medium density

Regimen: I shampoo once every two weeks with Mielle Babassu Oil Conditioning Sulfate-Free Shampoo and clarify once a month. I use Mielle White Peony Leave-in Conditioner as a refresher spray. I use Mielle Hair Milk every two to three days until I need to cleanse.

> "I started grow-ing my beard, so I thought that I would just let my hair grow out about seven months ago. To me it's a connection to my roots. I like to refer to what I'm doing right now as 'growing my crown.'"

—Robert Bjorn Taylor, bartender

Texture: 4b/4c, low poros-ity, coarse, thick

Regimen: I wash with all-natural cleanser but I don't really style. I just let it do what it does.

Chapter 11

CURLY MEN—

NOT JUST A BUZZ CUT

Throughout his life, Ryan Britton's curls have been a source of self-expression. He hated them as a kid, especially after puberty hit and gave him a head full of wild, tight 3b curls. His solution was to get monthly buzz cuts. "I wanted to avoid any unwanted attention," says Britton.

During his senior year of high school, as he got more in touch with his creative side, he decided to let his curls grow out. "This was something I was working on accepting anyway," he says.

In college, he shaved the back and sides and left the top long. Then he started growing it all out, trimming it only five times over the next decade. "My curls flowed down about eight inches below my shoulders. If you pulled on a strand, it would stretch to the pockets of my jeans."

He cut it off in 2007, and since then the father of four has experimented with various rockabilly and skater cuts—the wilder the better. "Not many folks have the hair or the guts to pull it off. It separates me from everyone else."

The Curl Revolution of the past two decades has extended to men, too. In fact, for many curly men, their struggle to embrace their texture has rivaled that of their female counterparts. Men, too, have grown up envying their peers with straight

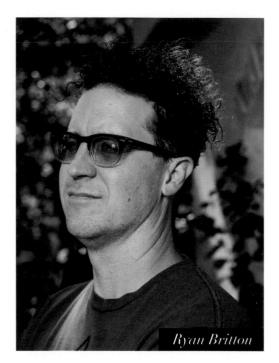
Ryan Britton

hair. They have been teased about their curls and coils. They struggle with frizz, dryness, and breakage. They've dealt with bad haircuts and the search for the right hair products.

In the past, the approach for many was to cut it short. But now, a growing number of men are taking advantage of their texture. Curl expert Shai Amiel of Capella Salon in Los Angeles says he has a growing clientele of curly men.

"Men, in general, are just going for it," Amiel says. "I think it's become so hip and trendy for us to embrace our natural texture. I see guys with long curly hair, short hair, and just about any length or color. A lot of my men really want to see what their hair will look like longer, but a lot of my men still love the big, rounded, messy, curly shapes."

Coily men, especially, are using their hair as a form of self-expression, rocking fades, twists, or big, luscious Afros.

Hair care advice for curly men is similar to suggestions for curly women: find a stylist or barber who knows how to work with texture and use products that work for your texture type.

If you aren't sure what to do, you'll get plenty of help from the growing number of male influencers with curls and coils who are inspiring and educating men about how to work with their texture. Vlogger Graham (who goes just by his last name) started his YouTube channel in 2014 because of the lack of "role models" for 3c/4a coily men. On his channel he offers how-tos and hair product reviews.

"When I started my curly hair journey, I had no idea what to use and which products work for my hair," says Graham. "It took me a long time to figure that out, and at some point I thought I would never find the right products. But now, almost three years after starting my YouTube channel, I know exactly what I like and what my hair needs."

Influencer Jor-El Caraballo created his

> " I was very nervous about how people would respond to this growing thing on my head. I realized my Afro is the perfect reflection of who I am, and people understand it."

—Jor-El Caraballoa, male natural hair influencer, founder of manemanblog.com

Texture: 4b, high porosity/ low porosity, coarse, thick

Regimen: I shampoo twice a week with Victory 2-in-1 Triple Threat Shampoo & Conditioner, Condition with Garnier Whole Blends Nourishing Conditioner with Avocado Oil & Shea Butter. Then, I rake in SheaMoisture Coconut & Hibiscus Curl & Style Milk and scrunch in Dove Men+Care Control Gel for extra control. I'll finish with Oyin Handmade Burnt Sugar Pomade.

> "I grew up thinking I had to wear it a certain way—short and trimmed. My hair reflects me getting out of my comfort zone and doing something I haven't done before. After being restrained for so many years, I'm letting it do its own thing. It's very reflective of my own personal journey. I had a strict upbringing. I moved to the city and cut loose."

—Warner King Washington II, artist and personal trainer

Texture: 4a/4b, low porosity, coarse, thick

Regimen: I use Hair Rules Shampoo and Conditioner, Hair Rules Leave-In Conditioner, and Hair Rules Styling Cream.

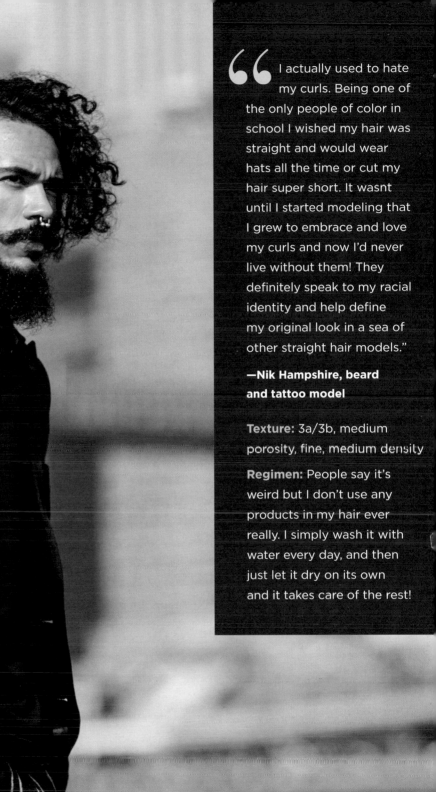

> "I actually used to hate my curls. Being one of the only people of color in school I wished my hair was straight and would wear hats all the time or cut my hair super short. It wasnt until I started modeling that I grew to embrace and love my curls and now I'd never live without them! They definitely speak to my racial identity and help define my original look in a sea of other straight hair models."

—Nik Hampshire, beard and tattoo model

Texture: 3a/3b, medium porosity, fine, medium density

Regimen: People say it's weird but I don't use any products in my hair ever really. I simply wash it with water every day, and then just let it dry on its own and it takes care of the rest!

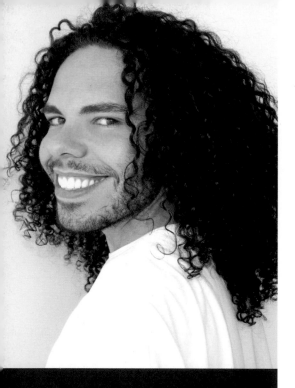

Mane Man online lifestyle guide to discuss everything from hair to shaving to men's health. Caraballo's website started after he decided to grow out his hair for the first time and experienced some emotional and physical changes. He wanted to create a place where men of all races could share their experiences and find support for both hair- and non-hair-related issues.

When he decided to grow out his 4b coils, he says, "I was starting from square one. It's been a constant evolution of learning what works. I have a much better idea of what works now, and have my core routine now."

That routine includes washing two times a week with 2-in-1 shampoo/conditioners and using a naturally derived conditioner with shea butter or coconut oil. He follows that with a leave-in conditioner and pomade. He adds a gel on humid days for more control.

One of NaturallyCurly's original male CurlTalkers was Jordan Pacitti, who discovered the site shortly after it launched. He started wearing his curls short in fifth grade—so short that his curls were nonexistent. He kept it that way until he moved away from home to study ballet at the American Ballet Theatre in New York City.

"It was the first time I felt that my hair was unique *and* accepted," Pacitti says.

But he still had to figure out how to care for his curls. "I had always had super-short hair so I never had any challenges *until* I started growing it out," he says.

For Caraballo, embracing his texture has been a big confidence builder. "I was very nervous about how people would respond to this growing thing on my head. I realize it's the perfect reflection of who I am."

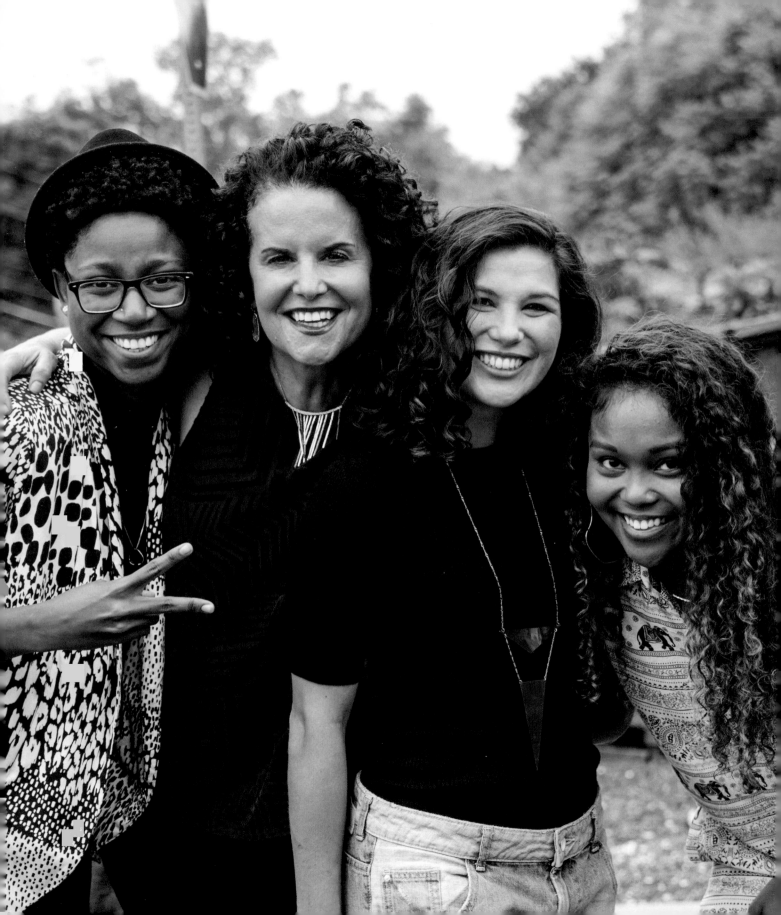

CONCLUSION

During a recent interview, a beauty editor asked me whether curly hair was now mainstream.

I thought about that question.

On the surface, she certainly had a point.

Natural hair is much more common than it used to be in pop culture—from the music industry to television shows. But it was still a major statement on *How to Get Away with Murder* when Viola Davis's Annalise Keating pulled off her wig to reveal her natural hair. After 20 seasons of *The Bachelor*—that cheesy cultural barometer—I can count the number of curly contestants on one hand—or at least the number of girls who wore their hair curly.

Models with curls and coils now can be found in ads for everything from J. Crew to Progresso Soup. But the Council of Fashion Designers of America still had to release racial diversity guidelines last year—nearly 10 years after the discussion started—to encourage diversity on the runway.

Products for texture occupy a growing amount of shelf space at stores like Target and Wal-Mart. But some of the largest companies still dedicate limited resources to the category—a fraction of their overall product offerings.

Every week, there's an event dedicated

to natural hair somewhere in the world. But at the largest professional beauty shows, many of the brands specializing in texture are tucked away in the back.

There are more salons than ever specializing in curly hair. But in most cities, it's still hard to find stylists who know how to work with texture.

The man at the flat iron kiosk at the mall still chases me down regularly, assuming that I must want to straighten my curls.

Veteran curl stylist Amie Zimmerman expressed it best in an essay she recently wrote for TheBigSmoke.com:

> **"Our culture says that curly-haired people are unhirable, untrustworthy, and unlovely. That people who choose to wear their hair curly are of a less desirable race or class, and that straight hair is an upgrade, a sign of wealth or at least upward mobility. That people who wear their hair natural are somehow making this radical social statement, bucking the standards of beauty, giving the finger to the Man."**

While Zimmerman calls her straight locks "unremarkable," she says that's not the case for most of the clients at XO Salon in Portland, Oregon.

> **"Their hair is weird and of note and fair game for comments from strangers when worn naturally. I hear these stories daily when I'm behind the chair, and although most of the time my clients aren't saying it that explicitly, it's the message they hear from a very young age."**

NaturallyCurly isn't going anywhere. There's still work left to do. And we look forward to the next chapter. We invite you to be a part of it.

ACKNOWLEDGMENTS

Neither NaturallyCurly nor this book would have happened without my cofounder and editor Gretchen Heber, who poured her passion and talent into the site and helped me with initial edits of the book. Many thanks to contributing writer Erica Metzger—who helped me shape the book when it seemed like an overwhelming endeavor. Special thanks to Christo of Christo Fifth Avenue, Anthony Dickey of Hair Rules Salon, The Devachan Salon, Cozy's Cuts for Kids and Lark Salon for opening up your salons to us for our photo shoots.

A huge thank you to Jimmy Treybig—high-tech icon and venture capitalist—who believed in our curly dream early on and provided invaluable business advice and encouragement. He helped us believe that our tiny hobby could become a multi-million-dollar business and invested time and money into NaturallyCurly.

Neither NaturallyCurly nor "The Curl Revolution" would be possible without our amazing NaturallyCurly team members, and all of the contributors who help us remain a leader in this industry.

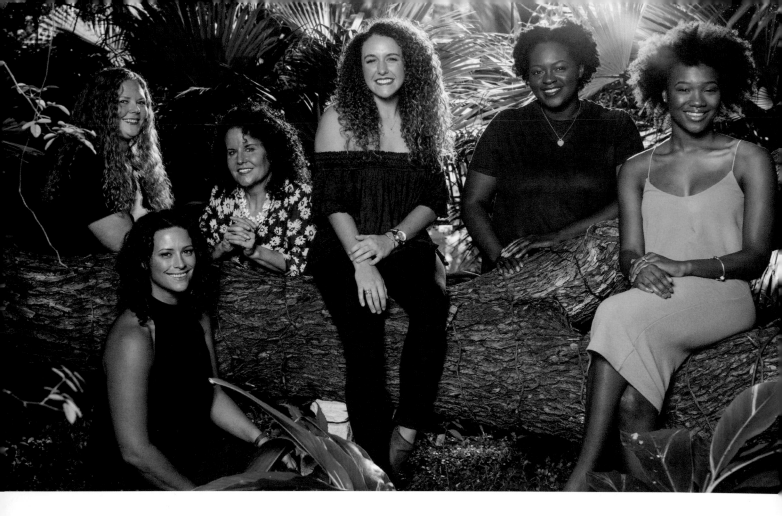

Thank you to our parent company, Ultra/Standard Distributors, for providing the resources that enabled us to hire the best for this book, including our amazing photographer Karston "Skinny" Tannis, who truly brought "curls to life" through his gorgeous photos.

Special thanks to Gregory and Heidi Kallenberg, who hosted the brunch where we hatched the idea for NaturallyCurly, and to Ben Friedman who suggested we start a web site after listening to our 45-minute bitch session.

My husband Jody, and curly daughter, Emma, deserve extra thanks for their support and patience throughout this process, which consumed much of my free time over the past year.

Finally, I want to thank my curly father, Jack, and straight-haired mother, Miriam—my curly father for contributing his genes and my straight-haired mother for cutting my hair into a pixie for the first 13 years of my life. They instilled me with the belief that anything and everything is possible.

CURLIPEDIA

*P*lopping? Co-wash? Pineappling? Curly hair care is full of bewildering lingo. Check out NaturallyCurly's glossary of hair care terms, including many terms created by our creative community.

Aloe Vera Gel: Obtained from the aloe vera plant, the benefits of aloe vera gel to your hair include improved detangling, increased moisture, scalp healing, remediation of dandruff, restoration of pH levels, decreased frizz, anti-inflammatory action for the scalp, and generation of hair growth.

Ammonium Laurel Sulfate: A harsh surfactant found in most shampoos. It is an ingredient that can cause the hair to become excessively dry after cleansing, so most curlies navigate toward cleansers with gentler cleansing agents.

Accordion Technique: Wash-and-go styling technique that produces well-formed, highly defined coils/curls. (Best if performed in the shower because it involves significant dripping.) Hair is first cleansed and conditioned. While soaking wet, a styling curl cream or curl gel is applied. As the head is titled in various angles, the hair—now weighted with water and styling product—is lowered into an open palm and gently pressed to the scalp repeatedly. Hair is typically air-dried afterward.

ACV (Apple Cider Vinegar): When apple cider vinegar is diluted with water, it can be used to restore a healthy pH balance to the hair and scalp. Additionally, an ACV will close the hair's cuticle, making it smooth with less frizz and provide ultimate shine. For an ACV, mix 1/4 cup of apple cider vinegar and 2 cups of water.

Armpit Length: Armpit length is when the ends of the hair on the back of the head reach a person's armpits (when stretched out).

Ayurvedic Regimen: This regimen uses all-natural Indian products to grow healthy, thick, long hair. Some of the products include but are not limited to the following: amla oil or powder, henna, neem, Vatika, brahmi, shikakai, and marshmallow root.

Baggy Method: The baggy method includes applying moisturizer and then covering the hair with a plastic bag to trap body heat for expedited product absorption into the hair's cuticle.

Banding: A styling technique used to inhibit hair shrinkage and thereby display more of the hair's actual length. The hair is gathered into one ponytail or several smaller ones, and then covered elastic bands are affixed snugly and progressively from the scalp area, one after the other, all the way down to the ends (or near the ends) of the hair. Several bands may be needed for each section, depending upon hair length. May be done on wet, damp, or dry hair. Bands are left in for a period of time or until the hair is dry (if banded while damp or wet).

Bantu Knots: A hairstyle created by carefully and precisely parting hair in small-to-medium sections, and then twisting the sections in one direction until they wrap into neat knots. The knots are often secured near the scalp with bobby pins or hairpins.

Big Chop: This is when a person decides to go natural and cut off all chemically relaxed hair. To Big Chop includes cutting the relaxed and significantly heat-damaged portions of the hair, leaving only the new-growth natural hair. Psychologically, this is often a time of major significance in one's journey from relaxed to natural hair.

Blowout: A blowout simply means styling your hair straight with a round brush as you blow it dry.

Bra-Strap Length: Bra-strap length is when the ends of your hair can reach the back of your bra strap upon extension.

Canopy: The canopy is the top layer of hair that is exposed to the elements most often, and is most prone to frizz.

Carrier Oil: This is an oil derived from plants and used to dilute essential oils before applying to the hair or body. Some popular carrier oils that curlies love include olive oil, avocado oil, sweet almond oil, grape seed oil, jojoba oil, and sunflower oil.

Castor Oil: Castor oil has the antibacterial and antifungal properties of ricinoleic acid, which can help prevent scalp infections that can cause hair loss. It is a humectant that contains fatty acids to nourish the hair and prevent dry scalp.

Clarify: Clarifying is the practice of thoroughly removing buildup from excess sebum, environmental elements, chlorine, and products from the hair. Clarifying shampoo and bentonite clay are among the most-often-used clarifiers.

Cleansing Conditioner: Cleansing conditioners are also known as co-wash conditioners. These products are formulated to lightly cleanse and moisturize the hair between clarifying treatments. They are moisturizing like conditioners, but contain surfactants that remove dirt and oil from the hair.

Clumping: Clumping happens when the strands of hair gather together to form bigger, chunkier curls.

Co-Wash: To co-wash is to use a conditioner to lightly cleanse and moisturize the hair between clarifying treatments. The term is short for "conditioner wash." Co-washes are used by curly-haired women who choose not to use shampoo as part of the Curly Girl Method or the No 'Poo Method.

Coconut Oil: An ingredient derived from coconuts with a molecular structure that easily penetrates the hair shaft. It has antifungal and antibacterial properties and is rich in vitamins and minerals.

Crown: The crown is the center region of the scalp atop the head. It tends to be sensitive, especially for those who are tender-headed.

Crunch: Crunch is the hard, crunchy feeling left in the hair by some gels when they dry, and can sometimes be scrunched out.

Curly Girl Method: The Curly Girl Method is a hair care method that disallows the use of shampoos and products containing silicones, as well as brushes, combs, or towels. This method is attributed to curly hair expert Lorraine Massey.

Deep Condition: To deep condition means using a thick product formulated with ingredients that penetrate the hair shaft to nourish between the cuticles, within the cuticle layers, and/or within the cortex. Deep conditioners generally require longer treatment time, which can be anywhere between 10 to 30 minutes based on manufacturer's instructions. The practice derives its name from the fact that it conditions the hair more deeply than normal daily conditioners.

Density: Density refers to how closely individual strands of hair are packed together on the scalp and ranges from low to high.

Diffuser: A diffuser is a blow-dryer attachment used to disperse the airflow over a larger area so the air doesn't disturb the hair's wave pattern or cause frizz while drying the hair. (Product type)

Dusting: Dusting is the slight trimming of hair in between haircuts.

Elongation: The process of loosening the curl pattern (and therefore "lengthening" the appearance of the hair) with products or techniques.

Emollient: Emollients are usually hydrophobic oils that form films on the surface of the hair, where they often act as anti-humectants or sealants. They are lubricants and provide increased slip (decreased drag) between adjacent hair strands, which makes detangling much easier.

Essential Oil: Essential oils are potent liquids derived from flowers and parts of many plants. They are known for their healing properties and aromatic scents that have therapeutic benefits, including maintaining a healthy scalp. Some essential oils for the hair are tea tree, rosemary, lavender, lemon, ylang ylang, chamomile, myrrh, basil, sage, and peppermint oil.

Extra Virgin Olive Oil (EVOO): Extra virgin olive oil is extracted through cold pressing, which uses only pressure to extract the oil. It is one of the four oils that penetrate the hair shaft. Many curlies use this to pre-'poo, deep condition, oil rinse, and seal.

Fine Texture: Fine hair is a hair type where each strand has a very small diameter and is very delicate and easy to damage.

Fatty Alcohol: Fatty alcohols are derived from natural sources and are often used as emollients in skin and hair care products. They give a smooth, soft feeling to the hair shaft by helping the cuticle to lie flat on the surface of the hair. Some fatty alcohols include lauryl alcohol, cetyl alcohol, myristyl alcohol, stearyl alcohol, cetearyl alcohol, and behenyl alcohol.

Flat Twists: A two-strand twist where the hair is twisted flat to the scalp, in cornrow fashion.

Fluff: The use of fingers or a pick to add volume and shape to curly and coily hair.

Fro: Afro

Frohawk: A hairstyle where the sides of an Afro are flattened to the scalp, either by smoothing and pinning or by shaving. The center hair is left high and free, in the shape of the distinctive mohawk.

Glycerin: A water-soluble conditioning alcohol that is an extremely effective moisturizer and humectant.

Hair Types: Hair typing is a system that classifies a person's hair texture based on curl pattern, density, width, and porosity, and helps to determine how she will care for and style her hair. Loose-wavy hair is type 2, curly hair is type 3, and coily hair is type 4. The sub classifications, from a to c, are based upon the diameter of the wave, curl, or coil.

Henna: Henna is an herbaceous shrub whose extracts are used to condition and safely color the hair. It is commonly used in India for cultural customs and for conditioning the hair.

Holy Grail: Holy Grail is a title given to the tried-and-true products that can be relied on to deliver consistently amazing results. Each person's Holy Grail products are different, as each head of hair is unique. Furthermore, a person's Holy Grail products may change over time.

Humectant: A humectant is an ingredient in moisturizing products that absorbs moisture from the air to transfer it to the hair. Some of the most commonly used humectants are honey, aloe vera, and glycerin.

Jamaican Black Castor Oil: This is an oil rich in Omega-9 acids that moisturizes the scalp to help with dry, brittle hair, hair breakage, dandruff, dry scalp, thinning hair, and alopecia. It can encourage hair growth. Black Castor Oil is made from the castor bean. The ash in Jamaican Black Castor results from roasting the beans and makes it more potent than regular castor oil.

Jojoba Oil: Jojoba oil is a non-greasy, moisturizing hair oil that is the most similar to the sebum produced by the sebaceous glands in your scalp.

Keratin: Keratin is a protein; it is the main building block of hair. Damage to the hair cuticle can lead to a loss of keratin, which can cause hairs to break. Keratin-containing hair care products can fill in gaps in the hair cuticle.

Leave-In Conditioner: A leave-in conditioner is a lightweight, watery product that is formulated to add moisturizing properties to the hair without the buildup of a regular conditioner. It derives its name from the fact that this conditioner is not rinsed out, but rather left on the head to work all day.

Line of Demarcation: During the time a person is transitioning from relaxed hair to natural hair, the line of demarcation is the point at which new hair growth meets old-growth, chemically relaxed hair. This "line" is particularly fragile and must be handled with extreme care to prevent the relaxed hair from breaking off.

Locs: A hairstyle whereby small sections of hair are twisted and over time, the strands become permanently secured. As locs grow, they can become quite long. This is one type of protective style.

L.O.C. Method: The L.O.C. Method stands for applying product in the following order: liquid or leave-in conditioner, oil, cream. Most naturals will either use water or a moisturizer, an oil, and a cream or butter. This will help to ensure long-lasting, moisturized hair between wash days. The technique was introduced by the founder of Alikay Naturals, Rochelle Graham.

Medium Texture: Hair with medium width consists of strands that are strong and elastic, and neither too thin nor too thick.

Mineral Oil: A mixture of simple hydrocarbon molecules of varying molecular weight derived from the petroleum-cracking process. Its molecular structure is very uncomplicated, extremely stable, and nonreactive. It is used in hair care products to seal moisture in.

Moisturizer: A moisturizing product that includes humectants, which are extremely hydrophilic molecules that use hydrogen bonding to attract and hold water molecules from the environment. Some examples of these types of ingredients are glycerin, propylene glycol, panthenol, honey, agave, and aloe vera.

Nappyversary/Nattyversary: The anniversary of the day one decided to "go natural" and to refrain from applying chemical straighteners (relaxers) to the hair.

No-'Poo Method: Removing from one's hair care regimen shampoo, products formulated with water-insoluble silicones, and products that require sulfates for proper cleansing.

Olive Oil: A heavier oil, olive oil contains vitamin A, vitamin E, and helps retain moisture.

Oil Rinsing: To rinse your hair with an oil after cleansing and before conditioning. To oil rinse, one adds a favorite oil to wet strands and leaves on the hair for about 5 minutes. This step helps to detangle and seal in extra moisture.

Paraben: Parabens are preservatives commonly used in cosmetic products.

Phthalate: Phthalates are a chemical group used in hair and skin products such as hair sprays, soaps, and shampoos. The most common phthalates used are dibutylphthalate (DBP), dimethylphthalate (DMP), and diethylphthalate (DEP). Phthalates are plasticizers (dispersants) that reduce brittleness/cracking/stiffness, allowing them to form a flexible film.

Pineapple: To gently gather the hair atop the crown with a hair tie to preserve curls for second-day hair.

Plopping: This method includes wrapping wet hair in a T-shirt or microfiber towel in order to quickly and gently absorb excessive water that would otherwise drip.

Polyquat: Polyquats (polyquaternium) are polymers (natural or synthetic molecules) frequently used in hair care products to provide conditioning benefits to the hair.

Porosity: Porosity is how easily hair is able to absorb and hold moisture and chemicals. There are varying degrees of porosity that curlies commonly use to classify hair: high porosity, medium porosity, and low porosity.

Pre-'Poo: This includes applying an oil or conditioner prior to shampooing to help the hair maintain necessary moisture during the drying shampoo process.

Product Junkie: A product junkie is a person who has a habit of buying more products than necessary due to new product releases, sales, and product-bandwagon tendencies.

Propylene Glycol: This is a humectant found in many personal care products, including shampoos, conditioners, leave-in conditioners, and styling products. It is known to be a very effective humectant.

Protective Style: This is style that does not expose the ends of the hair and is typically left unmanipulated for 2–4 weeks, primarily used to retain length.

Protein Treatment: A protein treatment deposits protein structures on the hair's cuticle in order to replace protein that was lost through manipulation, chemical processing, aging, and the hair becoming older. These tend to be strong, and while everyone's protein sensitivity is different, it is usually advised to incorporate a protein treatment into one's regimen no more than once a month. Some proteins include hydrolyzed wheat, hydrolyzed keratin, and hydrolyzed quinoa.

PVP: Polyvinylpyrrolidone (PVP) is a water-soluble polymer found in most gels. It is an excellent film former and is relatively inexpensive. The water solubility is extremely attractive to companies that wish to sell products to consumers who do not use shampoo or who use very mild shampoos, as it makes the gel easy to rinse.

Scrunching: To scrunch is to gently squeeze the hair upward from ends toward roots to encourage curl definition and remove gel crunch (aka "scrunch the crunch").

Sealing: Sealing is applying an oil or cream following a water-based moisturizer or leave-in conditioner. Essentially it is sealing moisture into the hair, with most of the focus being on the ends. The molecules in most butters/oils are too large to pass into the hair, so they stick to the outside of the shaft, trapping in the rich goodness of the moisturizer.

Shea Butter: Shea butter is derived from the nut of the shea tree and is rich in vitamins A and E. It restores moisture and prevents weather damage. It is useful for preventing dry scalp and does not clog pores. It is also a good tool for sealing the ends of the hair.

Shoulder-Length: Shoulder-length hair is hair that reaches the shoulders.

Shingling: A form of wash-and-go styling whereby a styling curl cream or curl gel is liberally applied section by section to clean, very wet hair. As the styling product is applied to each relatively small section of hair, the section is smoothed between the thumb and forefinger, in a downward motion from root to tip. The smoothing action, in combination with the styling product, immediately makes the coil/curl/wave pattern evident. The hair is then either air-dried or dried with the use of a hood dryer. Once dry, the hair can be gently fluffed for style.

Shrinkage: Shrinkage is when the hair retracts after washing or being exposed to moisture (humidity). During this state, the hair's true length is not apparent. To avoid this, some curlies will stretch their hair through twisting, braiding, and other styling methods. Hair experiences the most shrinkage in a wash-and-go style.

Silicate: Silicates are water-soluble inorganic minerals that are used as viscosity modifiers (thickeners).

Silicone: Silicones are (generally) non-water-soluble conditioning agents used in shampoos, rinse-off conditioners, intensive treatment conditioners, and leave-in conditioners where they reduce combing friction, provide an emollient effect, impart gloss, and reduce static charge between hair strands.

Slip: Slip refers to how lubricious a product makes hair feel after applying. The nickname is derived from the feeling of being "slippery" in one's hand. If fingers, comb, or brush can slip between hair strands with ease, the hair is said to have "great slip," and can be detangled more easily, with reduced risk of breakage.

Slippery Elm: The powered bark from the slippery elm tree is highly effective in hair care, especially for curlies, as it is an amazing natural detangler.

Sodium Lauryl Sulfate (SLS): Sodium lauryl sulfate is a surfactant cleanser found in most shampoos that creates a great lather for cleaning, but is extremely harsh and drying. Sodium lauryl sulfate (SLS) and sodium laureth sulfate (SLES) are known to be among the harshest surfactants due to their potential to be drying to the skin and hair.

Sulfate: "Sulfate" is a grouping term used to refer to any of a large number of sulfate-based surfactants that tend to be extremely harsh on curly hair, and therefore have been spurned by many curlies who have decided to forgo products with this ingredient. In response, many manufacturers now formulate products without this ingredient.

Surfactant: A surfactant is a detergent molecule that has one distinct portion that is polar and hydrophilic (water-loving), and one portion that is non-polar and hydrophobic (water-fearing). Surfactants are used in cleansing and conditioning products to remove buildup.

Tailbone Length: Tailbone length refers to hair that reaches one's tailbone.

Tea Tree Oil: Tea tree oil is a powerhouse oil that has antibacterial, antioxidant, and antiseptic properties. In the curly world, it is primarily used for scalp conditions such as seborrheic dermatitis, fungal conditions, and dandruff.

Teeny Weeny Afro (TWA): A teeny weeny Afro is a short hairstyle characterized by the inability to create a ponytail, because the hair is too short.

Transitioning: Transitioning is the process of growing out chemically straightened hair by not cutting the relaxed ends or cutting them slowly over time.

Twist Out: A twist out is when you intertwine two clusters of hair like a rope, allow it to set or dry, and then release the twists. People wear this style loose or coif it into updos.

Underlayer: The underlayer is the hair under the top, exposed layer.

Updo: An updo is a hairstyle worn up and not loose.

Wash-and-go: A styling method wherein one washes one's hair, applies moisturizer and/or styling products, and allows the hair to dry naturally, without stretching or otherwise manipulating the hair to obtain length or other styling attributes.

Wheat Protein: Wheat protein preparations are rich in unsaturated fatty acids; the preparations make hair shinier and easier to manage, and they also strengthen damaged hair.

Width: Width is the thickness of individual hair strands that range from fine to coarse.

INDEX

A

acceptance, 34, 37
accessories, 122, 203
actresses, 25, 227
Afro, 115, 132
Afrobella, 5
air-drying, 121, 193
alcohols, 82, 196
Almonte, Elizabeth, 62
aloe, 47, 181
Amiel, Shai, 193, 220
amino acids, 84
Atkinson, Sydney, 130

B

Bailey, Diane, 11, 144
balayage highlights, 179
banding, 110
Bantu knots, 111, 155
Barbie dolls, 209
Barrera, Andrea, 39
beauty standards, 15, 22, 25, 194, 206, 228
bedtime, 121, 193, 213, 217
beeswax, 192
Benu, Jamyla, 3
Big Afro, 194
Big Chop, 28, 129, 141
    case study, 146
    tips for, 145, 148
Billig, Talia, 32, 34
Black Earth Products, 10
Blackwell, Cassidy, 67
blogs, 5, 15, 34
blow-drying, 126, 193

blowouts, 17, 61, 169
Budge, Trac, 187
box braids, 153
braids, 114, 153
Branch, Miko, 11, 14
Branch, Titi, 11
brands. *see* products
Brazil, Asla, 188
breakage, 50, 131, 136, 197
brittleness, 47, 136, 195
Britton, Ryan, 219, 220
brushing, 126, 191, 216
buildup, 47, 78, 85
bullying, 22
bun drying, 118
butters, 84
buzz cuts, 219

C

Caires, Hortensia, 158
Camille Rose Naturals, 9
cancer patients, 199–200
Capella Salon, 220
Caraballo, Jor-El, 28, 34, 220, 221, 224
Carol's Daughter, 11, 19
Carter, Jane, 162
Carter, Rhea, 175
case studies
    Big Chop, 146
    coloring, 186
CG Method, 78
chemical treatments, 125, 126–127, 197
chemo curls, 199–200

children. *see* kids
Christo, 102, 160, 164, 189
clarifying, 78
cleansers, 74, 78, 91
cleansing
    after exercising, 201
    amount of shampoo, 216
    controversy, 77
    frequency, 78, 80, 191, 216
    and frizz, 191
    kids hair, 216
    'poo formulas, 77
    before styling, 120
clipping, 117, 199
clumping, 104, 105
coarse hair, 49
"cocktailing," 11, 17, 85
coconut cream recipe, 89
coily hair (type 4), 66–71
Collazo, Crystal, 60
Collier, Ayshia, 63
color fading, 185
coloring, 175–176
    all-over, 176
    case study, 186
    demi-permanent, 176, 178
    do-it-yourself tips, 183–185
    fantasy color, 181–182
    gray coverage, 179, 182–183
    highlights, 179–180
    inspiration, 184
    layering, 184
    lowlights, 183
    permanent, 179
    in salon *versus* home, 185

semi-permanent, 176, 178
   temporary, 178–179
combs, 37, 197, 213
conditioners, 74, 81
   adding heat, 47, 84
   combing in, 191
   daily, 82–83
   deep conditioning, 83–84,
      88, 89, 125, 196
   hall of fame products, 91
   for kids, 210
   leave-in, 47, 82–83, 120, 210
   moisturizing, 47
   and porosity, 45, 47
   with slip, 82, 213
confidence, 37, 224
connections, 34, 37
consultations, 165–166, 172
cortex, 44, 176, 178, 196
Council of Fashion Designers of
   America, 227
co-washing, 78
Cozy's Cuts, 214
Crook, Courtney, 152
Crowfoot, Keeley, 203
crunchy curls, 120
Cruz, Angelica, 140
cultural factors, 2, 5, 15, 25, 34
curl kabobs, 107
Curl Keeper, 11
curl lingo, 172
CurlMart, 16
Curlpopnhair website, 28
curlpopworld, 28
CURLS, 7, 16
CurlTalk, 2, 5, 15
   first-timers for natural curls,
      33
   texture changes, 51
   transitioning advice, 149
   traveling for expert cuts, 172
Curly Girl Collective, 28
Curly Girl (Massey), 78
Curly Hair Artistry, 41
curly hair (type 3), 60–65
CurlyNikki, 15

Curve Salon, 11
cuticle layers, 44, 178, 190, 191
cutting. *see* hair cuts

D
Da Costa, Diane, 194
damage. *see also* breakage
   blow-drying, 126
   chemical, 125, 197
   from chemotherapy, 200
   dryness, 195–196
   heat, 45, 125, 126, 193, 196
Davis, Michaela D., 30
Deardoff, Carley, 55
deep conditioning, 83–84, 88, 89,
   125, 196
Dellinger, Mahisha, 7, 16
Dennis, Richelieu, 11
density, 48–49
detangling, 82, 84, 197, 213–214
Devachan Salon, 11, 167, 179
DevaClips, 199
DevaCurl, 11, 18, 78, 166, 180
DevaCurl Academy, 165
"Deva Cut," 167
diameter. *see* texture
Diametrix, 170
Dickey, Anthony, 8, 9, 146, 169
diffusers, 37, 100
diversity, 227
dryness, 195–196
dry shampoo, 201
dusting, 159

E
e-commerce sites, 16
education, 34
elongation, 97
empowerment, 15, 25
endorsements, 15
entrepreneurs, 5, 9, 15
ethnicity, 2, 5, 25, 42
exercise, 201–203
experimenting, 81–82, 129, 145,
   207
extensions, 155

F
Facebook, 205
fairy knots, 198
fantasy color, 181–182
fatty alcohols, 82, 196
fine hair, 50
finger coils, 115
finger curls, 106
finishers, 92
finishing, 85
Flannigan, Alaina, 71
flat twists, 155
flaxseed, 15
float test, 48
formaldehyde, 127
forums, 2
Friedman, Cozy, 214, 215
frizz, 11, 34, 189–191
   accepting, 193
   air-drying, 193
   beauty of, 194
   emergency kit for, 193
   fabrics to avoid, 193
   hydration and, 191–192
   over cleansing, 191
   product application, 192
   products for, 192
   touching curls, 193
frohawk, 151, 178
Frozen, 209

G
Gaspard, Natasha, 25, 68
genetics, 44
glycerin, 84, 120
going natural, 129. *see also* Big
   Chop; transitioning hair
   acceptance, 131
   reasons for, 131, 132
   versatility, 131–132
   where to start, 132, 136
Gomes, Daniela, 18, 132, 137
Graham, 220, 224
GrahamsNaturalCurls, 224
grass-roots movement, 9
gray hair, 179, 182–183, 186

green tea vinegar rinse, 88
"Grow-Out Challenge," 131

H

hair cuts, 159–160. *see also* Big
    Chop; stylists
    "Carve & Slice," 166, 168
    "chemical haircut," 17
    combination wet/dry, 168
    consultations, 165–166
    "Deva Cut," 167
    dry cutting, 167–168
    and frizz, 191
    pictures of, 166, 174
    pyramid head, 199
    regular trims, 50, 139, 159,
      195, 200
    shrinkage, 17
    on straightened hair, 169
    tangle-free styles for kids,
      210
    techniques, 166–167
    wet cutting, 168, 170
hair follicles, 44
hair growth, 50, 145
hair loss, 197, 200
hair meet-ups, 34, 37
Hair Rules (Dickey), 9
hair shaft, 44, 176
hairspray, 121
hairstyles, 2, 97–119
    bans in schools, 18
    fitness-friendly, 203
    how-to videos, 96
    professional looks, 18
    techniques, 95–96
    tightness, 197
    tips, 120
    tools, 96
    for transitioning hair, 148,
      152
hair types. *see* types
hair vitamins, 92, 198
Hampshire, Nik, 223
Harbinger, Shari, 94, 165, 179,
    199

head wraps, 155
heat
    with conditioning, 47, 84
    damage, 45, 125, 126, 193,
      196
    for fine hair, 50
    protectants, 125–126, 196
heat-free curls, 153
Heber, Gretchen, 34
henna, 180–181
highlights, 179–180
Holy Grail, 6, 22, 90
homemade treatments, 87–89
Honeghan, Shellyann, 143
honey, 84
hot rollers, 17
humectants, 82, 84, 192
humidity, 17, 34, 120, 190
hydration, 45, 47, 191–192

I

ideas. *see* inspiration
influencers, 15, 28, 74, 175, 182,
    220
information sources, 34
inspiration, 34, 184, 214
Instagram, 33, 34, 172

J

Jenkins, Alexzandra, 36
Jessicurl, 12, 15
Johnson, Ashley, 64
Johnson, Candice, 151
jojoba, 47

K

Kahkoska, Jessica, 56
keratin, 44, 176, 182
keratin treatments, 126–127
kids
    detangling, 213–214
    messages heard by, 207,
      209–210
    name calling, 15, 16, 22, 34,
      35, 205, 206

    parents attitudes, 207,
      209–210
    products, 92, 214
    role models for, 206, 207
    straight-haired parents, 209,
      214
    tangle-free styles, 210
    teaching styling techniques,
      207, 209, 210
    touching hair, 210
    weekend regimens, 211, 213
knot out, Bantu, 111, 155
knots, 82, 198
knowledge, 34
Kwamya, Julia, 70

L

lanolin, 192
Laws-Phillips, Tauri, 134
Leal, Leticia, 54
leave-in coconut cream, 89
leave-in conditioners, 47, 82–83,
    120, 210
length, 50
LeYanna, Tierra, 66
locs, 155
Logue, Cara, 57
Lopez-Mays, Tiffany, 142
Lowe, Gia, 79
Luciano, Layla, 201

M

males. *see* men
Mane Man, 34, 224
Mane Moves Media, 25
Marshall, Morgan, 65, 95
Massey, Lorraine, 11, 78, 167
Mazzarino, Joey, 209
McGuinty, Jessica, 12, 15, 22
McLeod, Kayla A., 153
media images, 15, 25, 209, 214
medulla, 44, 176
meet-ups, 34, 37
melanin, 44, 182
Meline, Nicole, 202
men, 218, 219–225

microfiber towels, 37, 193
Mini Chop, 141
Miss Jessie's, 14
models, 227
moisture. *see* hydration
moisturizers, 45, 47
moisturizing deep conditioner recipe, 88
Montalto, Diane M., 58
Moody, Maranda, 161
movies, 25, 209
Muppets, 209
Musgrave, Scott, 41

N

Nash, Natasha, 133
NaturallyCurly
    product hall of fame, 90–92
    texture-typing system, 42, 45
    website launch, 2, 5, 9
natural oils, 191
negative messages, 25, 136, 148, 194, 207
new growth, 136, 145, 148, 200
nicknames, 15, 16, 22, 34, 35, 205
nighttime regimen, 121, 193, 213, 217
no-'poo routines, 78
nutrition, 197

O

Ogg, Shana, 177
oils, 47, 83, 84, 92, 196
Olaye, Iyore M., 146
olive oil, 84
ombre, 180
Ortega, Nicole, 26
Ouidad, 10, 14, 22, 104, 166

P

Pacitti, Jordan, 224
Pallante, Rachel, 59
panthenol, 84
Patterson, Erica, 157

P/DMAPA Acrylates Copolymer, 126
peppermint pre-'poo recipe, 88
perceptions, 194, 206
perm rods, 153
personal journeys, 6, 22, 25, 28, 145
Pettway, Jessica, 211
pillowcases, 37, 193, 213
pin curls, 106
pineapple, 112
Pintrest, 214
Pintura highlights, 179, 180
plopping, 96, 108
polymers, 126
ponytails, 110, 203
pool hair, 203, 216–217
pop culture, 25, 209, 214, 227
Pope, Jamila, 23, 129
porosity, 45, 47, 48, 178, 190
"Praying Hands" Method, 192
pre-'poo, 84, 88
prettiness, 33
Price, Kay, 150
Price, Lisa, 11, 19
The Princess Diaries, 25
"product junkies," 77
products
    application, 120, 191, 192
    buildup, 47, 78, 85
    hall of fame, 90–92
    homemade, 87–89
    lines, 11, 16, 17, 214, 227–228
    protein-based, 47, 84, 196
    selection, 74, 77
professional image, 18
protection
    heat, 125–126, 196
    nighttime, 121
    swimming, 203
protein-based products, 47, 84, 196
"psycurology," 165
Pyles, Kennett N., 75
pyramid head, 199

Q

Quaternium 70, 126

R

race. *see* ethnicity
rake and shake, 104
Raposo, Walki, 61
Redken line, 28
refreshers, 91, 121, 122, 201
regimens, 73–74
regrowth, 184, 200
relaxed hair, 6, 11, 131, 136
relaxers, 11, 17, 126–127, 131
revitalizers, 121
rinses, 78
Robinson, Paix, 225
Rodriguez, Monique, 217
Rojas, Ada, 24
roller sets, 119, 126
run and swift, 102

S

salons, 11, 165, 214
satin pillowcases, 37, 121, 193, 213, 217
scalp health, 141
scarves, 155
scrunching, 98, 120
Seaborn, Emma, 93
sealing, 83, 196
seasonal issues, 196
second-day hair, 121–122
sectioning curls, 120
self-confidence. *see* confidence
self-expression, 28, 220
shampoo. *see* cleansing
shea butter, 180
SheaMoisture, 11
shingling, 110
shrinkage, 11, 17, 168, 195
silicones, 85, 192
single-strand knots, 198
skip curls, 107
sleeping. *see* nighttime regimen
slip, 82, 213

slip 'n slide test, 48
Smaster method, 97
Snowymoon's moisture treatment, 87
social connections, 34, 37
social media, 1, 15, 18
Sparks, Jordin, 38
SSKs. *see* single-strand knots
Stallion, Hazel M., 178
standard of beauty, 15, 22, 25, 194, 206, 228
Starks, Tylur, 135
Stephens, Janell, 43
Stevens, Monica, 76
stigmas, 18
straightening
    blow-drying, 126
    damage from, 122, 125
    deep conditioning, 125
    to fit in, 17, 18, 25
    frequency, 125
    heat free alternatives, 126
    stretching before, 126
    temperature, 125–126
strength, 49
styles. *see* hairstyles
styling products. *see* products
stylists, 37
    consultations, 165–166, 172
    lingo, 172
    making clients feel good, 174
    portfolio, 172
    saying no to clients, 174
    teaching clients, 174
    training, 18, 160, 165, 172
    traveling distance to, 173
    word of mouth, 170
Sugar, Lisa, 31
sulfates, 77, 78, 185, 196
Sullivan, Cynthia, 154
super mayo deep-conditioning treatment, 89
super-soaker method, 105
swimming, 203, 216–217

T
Tamborra, Mary, 171
Tattooz, Tiffany, 37
Taylor, Robert B., 218
Teele, Myleik, 124
teeny weeny afro, 141, 148
Tendrils Salon, 11
texlaxing, 127
texture, 2. *see also* types
    appreciation, 37
    changes over lifespan, 51
    changes with hair growth, 145
    uniformity, 42
Textured Tresses (Da Costa), 194
TextureMedia, 15
texturizers, 126–127
thickness. *see* texture
thin hair, 50
Thompson, Kissa, 46
Thompson, Maria, 139
tools, 37, 92, 96
Torch, Jonathan, 11
touching curls, 121, 193, 210
towels, 37, 193
transitioning hair
    community advice, 149
    length of process, 139
    protective styling, 139, 153
    styles, 139, 148, 153
    stylist visits, 139
    taking it slowly, 136, 139
treatments, homemade, 87–89
trends, 16, 17
trial and error, 81, 129, 166, 192
triangle head, 199
trimming. *see* hair cuts
Trucks, Toni, 25, 29
Tubman, Nyema, 11
turbans, 155
tutorials, 126
TWA. *see* teeny weeny afro
Twilight Saga, 25
Twine, Nancy, 123
twirling, 106
twists, 95, 114, 155

Tyler, Storm, 138
types
    coily hair (type 4), 66–71
    curly hair (type 3), 60–65
    wavy hair (type 2), 54–59
typing systems, 42, 45, 53

U
updos, 155

V
Vasquez, Isabella, 28, 163
Vidal, Tyesha, 27
vitamins, 92, 198
volumizers, 48, 50

W
Waajid, Taliah, 10
Walker, Andre, 42
Walker, Elizabeth, 69
Walker, Erin, 156
Walton, Nikki, 15
Ward, Carla, 216
washing. *see* cleansing
Washington, Warner K., II, 222
wash 'n go, 111
wavy hair (type 2), 54–59
weather. *see* humidity
Wheatfall-McIver, Caydence, 208
width. *see* texture
wigs, 141, 155
Wilson, Marrisa, 128
working out, 201–203
World Natural Hair, Health and Beauty Show, 10
Wright, Tanya, 4, 5

Y
yogurt hair mask, 87
YouTube, 126, 210, 214, 220
Yursik, Patrice, 5, 20, 21–22

Z
Zimmerman, Amie, 228

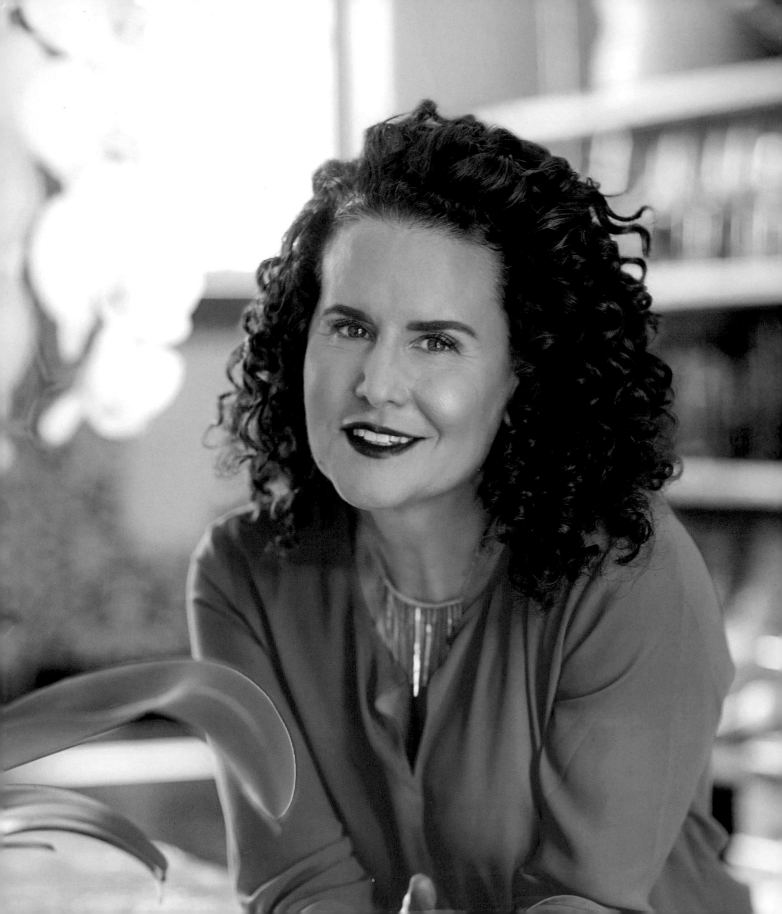

ABOUT THE AUTHOR

Named one of the 50 Most Influential People in the Multicultural Market by *Women's Wear Daily* in 2015, Michelle Breyer is a visionary entrepreneur who took a personal frustration over out-of-control curls and built it into one of the largest media platforms for hair. What started as a hobby for the former award-winning newspaper reporter now includes a consumer facing content and commerce web site, a popular lifestyle blog, and a market research division. NaturallyCurly's community now spends several billion dollars each year on hair care.

Michelle has consulted with companies both large and small to help shape their strategies for coils, curls, and waves, whether it be developing the right products or communicating effectively with the consumer. Michelle has shared her message of empowerment with other female entrepreneurs, inspiring them to channel their own passions into successful careers.

Michelle lives in Austin, Texas, with her husband, Jody, and curly daughter, Emma.

Photography by Brio Yiapan

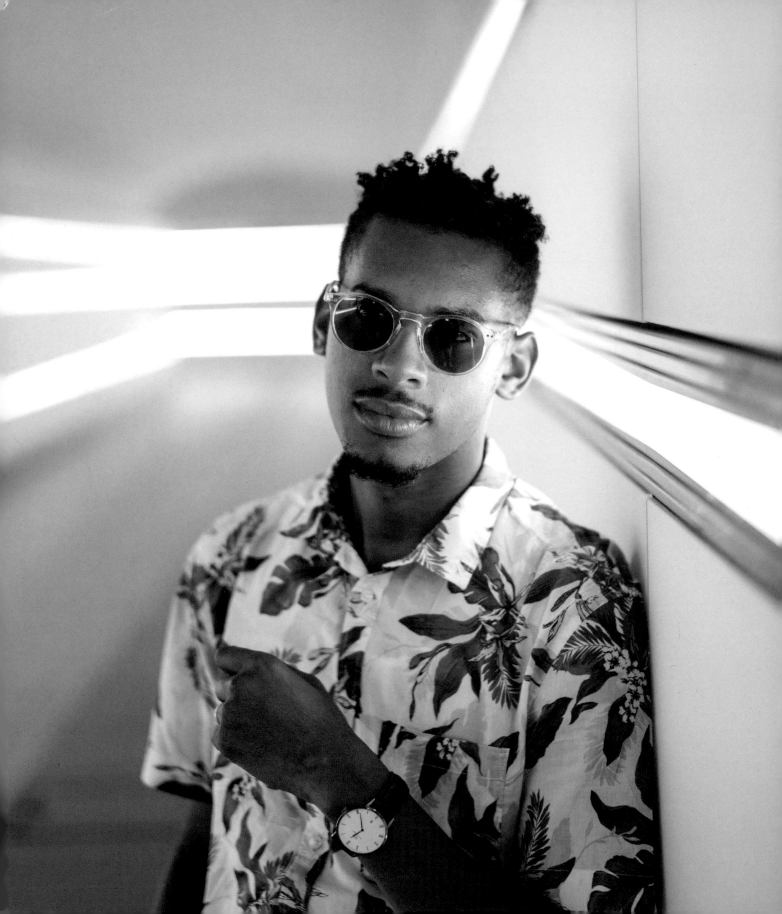

ABOUT THE PHOTOGRAPHER

Karston "Skinny" Tannis is a photographer specializing in environmental portraiture, lifestyle, and fashion photography. Karston uses his personality to engage with his subjects, capturing honest moments that resonate with viewers.

Hailing from Brooklyn, New York, Karston can be found roaming the streets of Soho or abroad in search of interesting styles and personalities while spreading positive vibes all around. For more information please visit www.karstontannis.com | @SkinnyWasHere.